GLOBAL HEALTH RESEARCH IN AN UNI WORLD

ETHICS CASE STUDIES FROM AFRICA

Gemma Aellah, Tracey Chantler, P. Wenzel Geissler

This page intentionally left blank

CABI
Nosworthy Way
Wallingford
Oxfordshire OX10 8DE
UK

CABI
745 Atlantic Avenue
8th Floor
Boston, MA 02111
USA

A catalogue record for this book is available from the British Library, London, UK.

Library of Congress Cataloging-in-Publication Data

Names: Aellah, Gemma, author. | Chantler, Tracey, author. | Geissler, Wenzel,
author. | C.A.B. International, publisher.
Title: Global health research in an unequal world : ethics case studies from
Africa / Gemma Aellah, Tracey Chantler, P. Wenzel Geissler.
Description: Oxfordshire, UK ; Boston, MA : CABI, 2016. | Includes
bibliographical references and index.

Commissioning editor: David Hemming
Editorial assistant: Emma McCann
Production editor: James Bishop

This page intentionally left blank

FOREWORDS

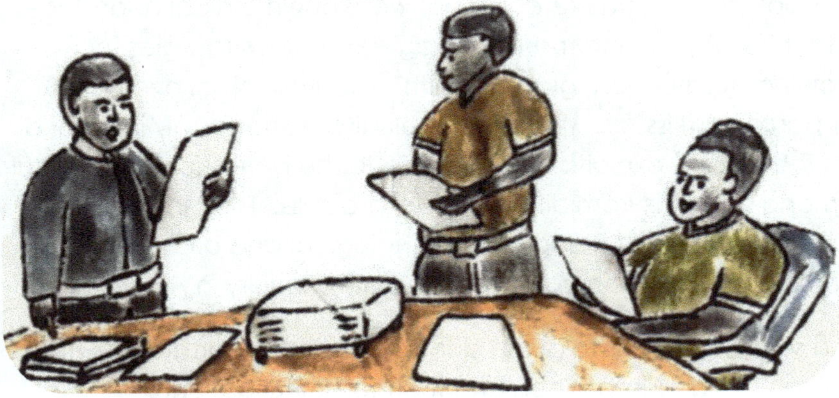

'WHAT DO YOU THINK ABOUT THIS BOOK?', 'NO, WHAT DO *YOU* THINK?'

PROFESSOR IRUKA N. OKEKE

IBADAN, NIGERIA, AUTHOR OF 'DIVINING WITHOUT SEEDS THE CASE FOR STRENGTHENING LABORATORY MEDICINE IN AFRICA' (2011)

I have spent most of my scientific career working trans-continentally between West Africa and the US and Europe as both an African and a Northern researcher. I have so many times been surprised, shocked and even stumped by the plethora of ethical challenges that emerge when individuals from vastly different backgrounds, with uneven but limited access to resources, study African life, death and disease. Several excellent resources for ethical reflection and training exist but too few address situations that are specific to Africa. Of those that do, most are too extensive or too specialized to be accessible to biological and clinical scientists. This single volume fills these critical gaps. By assembling this collection of thought-provoking case studies, the authors have skillfully constructed a resource that can be used in its entirety, or in a modular fashion, to guide thought and discussions around ethical issues of varying complexity. This book will become indispensable to individuals that work on, or engage with, experiments that are performed in or on Africa but which may be fully or partly conceived, conducted or interpreted elsewhere on the globe.

In the many case studies, the authors fearlessly point out misconceptions of Africans that predominate in the West, as well as African misconceptions of Euro-Americans. They illustrate that power is often tied to economics but that other resources can be similarly empowering. They prod researchers to think about and air inequalities associated with resource distribution, institutional support, compensation and career advancement of different actors within collaborations. This is not a manual for 'solving' ethical problems. Perhaps one of the most important lessons the book will teach those who seek to answer biological questions or solve clinical problems is that while ethical challenges should be identified, acknowledged and even mitigated against, many cannot easily be fixed.

Multiple case studies in this workbook go beyond sketching out well-known ethical quandaries to force readers or discussants to think beyond internationally agreed-upon strategies for addressing some issues. The growing literature on 'global health' research ethics overly focuses on patient or volunteer participant issues. While this book also leans heavily in favor of clinical trial scenarios, it extends the patient exploitation discourse to the professional, personal and institutional relationships among scientists from different backgrounds. Thus, in addition to medical researchers, this book will be of use to ecological, psychological and archeological researchers, indeed anyone who is engaged in so-called collaborative inquiry in Africa.

Each case is accompanied by a set of questions to guide discussions, helpful facilitator's notes and suggestions for further reading. The discussion tools and the thoughtful optional academic background section will be indispensable to biomedical research leaders who are, in general, not professional ethicists but need to formulate discussion questions and guide others to think about them. The mix of 'grassroots' and 'managerial' examples means that African and Western researchers can refer again and again to case studies as they advance or change roles in biomedical research. This resource should also be used by those that do not necessarily engage in transnational research but who study or reflect on its outcomes. Such individuals will include those conducting systematic reviews of the biomedical literature, teaching in 'global health' curricula, working in African health and educational institutions, or making decisions about research funding and publication.

PROFESSOR NELSON K. SEWANKAMBO

MBCHB, MSC, M.MED, FRCP, DOCTOR OF LAWS, HONORIS CAUSA, PRINCIPAL OF MAKERERE UNIVERSITY COLLEGE OF HEALTH SCIENCES, UGANDA

Many books on ethics are out there but this volume occupies a very special place. It is a great teaching and learning resource that is a must read and will be appealing to a large and varied audience: students who are training in health research, junior and senior indigenous and foreign researchers who engage or plan to engage in health research in Africa or in similar environments around the world, research administrators and managers, members of community advisory boards, research participants and the enlightened community members who wish to learn more about research ethics. It is easy to read and provides a bridge for moving from ethics regulations and rules to the realities and challenges of practicing ethics in the field. When I started reading it I could not stop and had to push aside many other commitments I had to do.

This new volume brings fresh thinking and emphasis in the field of relational ethics, from a social science perspective and grounded in fictionalised case studies from Africa. It relates very well to real life challenging field experiences encountered in research in Africa and yet it challenges one's thinking and promotes critical reflection. The cases cited are loaded with intriguing questions that the busy researcher or the less initiated individuals may just brush over and miss the real messages embedded in the case. As you scratch deeper you soon realise the richness of the cases and cannot help but to share these with peers and students or those in your research team.

Every passing year new ethics challenges emerge that remind us of the need to keep thinking and reflecting on these challenges because the field is not static. Books like this one originating in cases from Africa will in due course enable African researchers to play a more active and less passive role in debates on priority ethics issues that affect them and thus bring an African voice and experiences to inform these debates. In so doing they will contribute more meaningfully to advancing the field.

SIR BRIAN GREENWOOD

CBE, FRS, FMEDSCI, PROFESSOR OF CLINICAL TROPICAL MEDICINE, LONDON SCHOOL OF HYGIENE AND TROPICAL MEDICINE, UK

Clear general principles have been established to guide the ethical conduct of clinical research wherever this is conducted, but these may not help when detailed, practical decisions on what to do have to be made. This is especially the case in low income countries where there are many day-to-day challenges facing those who consider volunteering for inclusion in a research project. In such situations, should volunteers be paid for inclusion in a study and, if so, how much; should medical care be provided just to the volunteer or also to their family; how much autonomy should a woman have to make a decision about volunteering herself or her children for inclusion in a trial; how can confidentiality between volunteers and staff living in close contact with them in their community be maintained?

Frequently, there is no correct answer to such questions but, nevertheless, decisions have to be made. These are often guided by the prior experience of a senior member of the research team who knows the community well, but such a person may not be available and there are few other sources of help for researchers experiencing some of these challenges for the first time. This book aims to fill this gap and does so very successfully. Using a series of case studies, accompanied by evocative paintings by Johnson Ondiek, the authors provide examples of some of the common problems met by researchers working in low income settings and use these as the basis for discussion groups. In many cases, the correct course of action to follow is not obvious and the questions posed should elicit a lively debate.

It is clear that the case examples have been chosen by authors with extensive practical experience of dealing with the kind of problems faced every day by researchers in the developing world and they immediately strike a chord with the writer based on his own experience of conducting research in Africa. The book aims to raise awareness among mid-career researchers and students of some of the ethical challenges of conducting research in low income settings but reading these case stories may also cause more senior researchers to ponder on some of the decisions that they may be required to make. This is an important and original contribution to a neglected area that will be of value to many concerned with conducting clinical trials in poorly resourced communities whilst at the same time trying their best to maintain the highest standards of research ethics.

PREFACE

Conducting good, ethical global health research is now more important than ever. Increased global mobility and connectivity mean that in today's world there is no such thing as 'local health'. How we experience the effects of disease may be shaped by our particular social and political-economic circumstances, but the sick in one part of the world and the healthy in another are connected through economics, politics, media, and imagination, as well as by the infectiousness of disease. Global health research carried out through transnational collaboration is one crucial way in which people from far-flung geographic regions relate to each other. Good global health research, and the relationships it creates, therefore, concerns us all.

This book is a collection of fictionalized case studies of everyday ethical dilemmas and challenges often encountered in the process of conducting global health research in Africa where the effects of global, political and economic inequality are particularly evident. Our aim is to create a training tool which can begin to fill the gap between research ethics guidelines and their implementation 'on the ground'. The case studies, therefore, focus on everyday or 'relational' ethics: ethical actions and ideas that emerge through relations with others in context, rather than in universal principles or abstract regulations.

The fictional case studies are based on stories and experiences collected by a group of anthropologists who have worked with leading transnational medical research organizations across Africa over the past decade. The stories have been anonymised, combined with each other, and substantially altered in order to provide 'stumbling stones' to start discussions, without naming real places or situations.

As a collection, these stories offer a flexible resource for training across a variety of contexts, such as medical research organizations, universities, collaborative sites, and NGOs. We hope they will encourage global health researchers to think – and talk – about their everyday experiences and practices, and about ethics, in a new light.

AUTHORS:
GEMMA AELLAH
TRACEY CHANTLER
P. WENZEL GEISSLER

ADDITIONAL CONTRIBUTIONS:
BIRGITTE BRUUN
LUISA ENRIA
ANN H. KELLY
SHELLEY LEES
PHILISTER A. MADIEGA
FERDINAND OKWARO
FRANCESCA RAPHAELY

ILLUSTRATIONS:
JOHNSON A. ONDIEK

The authors and contributors to this book collaborated between 2005 and 2015 in the Anthropologies of African Biosciences Research Group

www.africanbiosciences.wordpress.com

AFFILIATIONS

Gemma Aellah is Research Officer at the Royal Anthropological Institute and a PhD researcher at the London School of Hygiene and Tropical Medicine

Tracey Chantler is Research Fellow at the London School of Hygiene and Tropical Medicine

P.Wenzel Geissler is Professor of Social Anthropology at the University of Oslo, Norway and part-time Director of research at University of Cambridge
p.w.geissler@sai.uio.no

ACKNOWLEDGEMENTS

We would like to thank the institutions, researchers and research participants across Africa who generously allowed us to learn from their experiences. Although the case studies are fictional, we hope that they all recognise the kind of situations described and see them as fair representations of their experiences.

We greatly appreciate the feedback that we received from scientists, ethicists, clinicians, fieldworkers, technical and administrative staff, community advisory board members, students, ethicists, and others, when we presented this project and piloted some of the stories with audiences in Kenya (Kenya Medical Research Institute, Ministry of Health), Norway (University of Oslo), Tanzania (National Institute for Medical Research), and the UK (London School of Hygiene and Tropical Medicine).

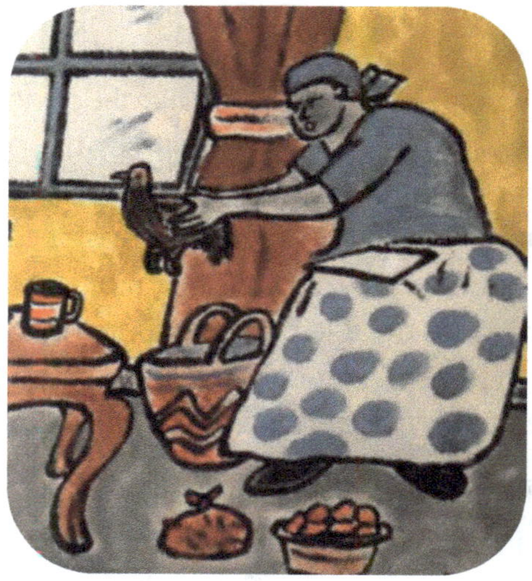

ASANTE SANA, THANK YOU, TAKK

We warmly thank our advisor, Dr John Vulule from the Kenya Medical Research Institute, for his support and guidance throughout this project, and some of the collaborative research that preceded it. Many thanks are also due to our illustrator Johnson A. Ondiek. As an artist who is also a practising African clinical researcher himself, his cloth paintings bring colour and life to our stories. All artwork is copyrighted to Johnson Alouch Ondiek at jaoarts@yahoo.com Thanks, finally, to Francesca Raphaely who not only proofread the manuscript but also added many a useful comment and query and in the process significantly improved the outcome.

Funding

This project, like much of the preceding research that informed our thinking, has been made possible through funding from the Leverhulme Trust (Research Leadership Award, PW Geissler, F/02 116D) and the Wellcome Trust (e.g., Geissler, GR077430; Chantler R087667). Gemma Aellah's PhD research was funded by Geissler's Leverhulme Trust Research Leadership Award, and a small grant from the British Institute of East Africa. The editorial work and the open access publication of the book were supported by the Wellcome Trust (098492/Z/12/Z).

Supported by wellcometrust

The Leverhulme Trust

CONTENTS

CONTENTS

FINDING YOUR WAY AROUND THE BOOK

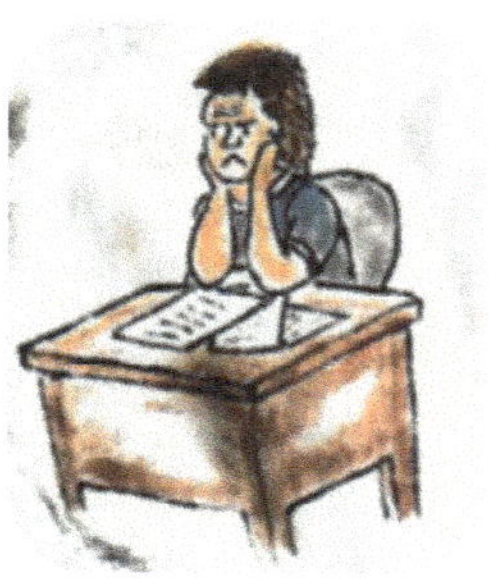

JUDY WONDERED WHERE TO START

The first part of this book is a short introduction to relational ethics, followed by a collection of **42** training case studies for global health researchers. We have divided the collection into four sections, each with a brief introduction to the section theme. Each section focuses on the different types of relationships that characterize the practice of global health research:

1. Researcher - participant relationships
2. Community and family relationships
3. Institutional relationships
4. Staff relationships

Each training case study comprises:

a. An introductory sheet for the training facilitator
   This includes a learning objective, keywords, and a commentary on the core ethical dilemmas that the story addresses.
b. A group handout
   This includes the story, an illustration, questions to prompt discussion and suggestions for further reading. Many of the case studies also include ideas for group activities.

A full list of case studies indexed by learning objective and keyword is provided at the end of the book.

The collection of case studies is followed by guidance on how to use the training case studies. We provide detailed advice on group use using the case **Helping hand** as an example; a template form to help facilitators prepare for a training session; and a list of additional resources such as key journals and websites. We also discuss insights from our own experiences of piloting the case studies with different groups in Africa and Europe.

The second part of this book provides a more in-depth discussion of the key perspectives informing our approach, an analysis of the context of transnational medical research in Africa, and an outline of what we believe anthropology and the social sciences can offer.

TRAINING CASE STUDY SECTIONS

1. RESEARCHER-PARTICIPANT RELATIONSHIPS

This collection of training case studies concerns issues arising out of direct interactions between researchers and study participants. The stories mainly focus on questions of 'good clinical practice' such as informed consent, coercion and participants' understanding of study protocols, but also include a consideration of both personal moralities and relationships. They include, for example, accounts of friendship between researchers and participants, as well as exploring how research staff introduce themselves, develop ongoing rapport, and balance their personal and professional identities. Some of the case studies explore particularly difficult issues relating to structural inequalities and working with poor populations such as how to deal with participants' hunger and post-research responsibilities for participants' welfare.

2. COMMUNITY AND FAMILY RELATIONSHIPS

This collection focuses on what is commonly known as 'community engagement'. It includes stories about rumours, the challenges of working with community advisory boards, and 'therapeutic misconception', where research activities are confused with treatment programmes. It also includes stories about the role of gender and family relationships in research participation. In contrast with Section 1, the relationships in this section are to do with kinship and community, and lie outside the immediacy of personal interactions between a research participant and a researcher.

3. INSTITUTIONAL RELATIONSHIPS

This collection covers collaborative relationships between governments, ministries of health, health facilities, research funders, and researchers. The stories deal with the various mandates, responsibilities and aims of different institutions, their unequal access to resources and expertise, and the relative importance of local experience and global scientific scope. Misunderstandings and tensions can arise between these groups of people who may have different aims, limitations and responsibilities. Many stories in this section invite discussion on the wider relationships between and across countries involved in global health research.

4. STAFF RELATIONSHIPS

This collection explores the kind of workplace relations characteristic of transnational collaboration. It includes stories of scientific co-operation between researchers from different institutions and backgrounds, as well as between different organizational levels and hierarchies; tensions that arise from unequal access to education, resources and decision-making; accusations of nepotism and corruption; experiences and perceptions of 'culture clash'; and simple misunderstandings.

INTRODUCTION

REGULATORY VERSUS RELATIONAL ETHICS

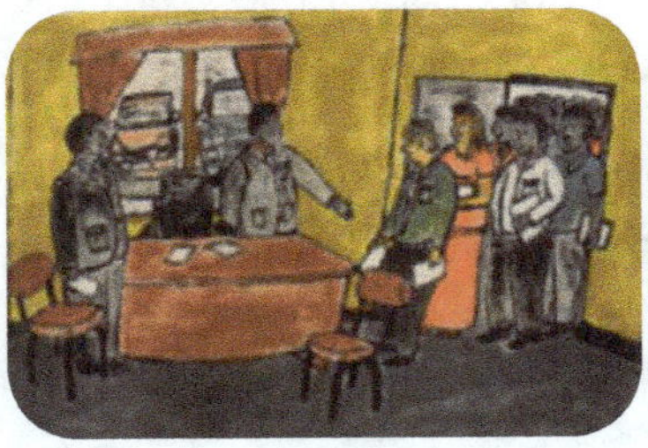

RESEARCH IS ABOUT PEOPLE

Global health research is not just about blood samples, laboratory technologies, data capture and translating evidence into health policy. It is about people. More specifically it is about relationships between people. It is the relationships between funders, government staff, local and international scientists, fieldworkers, research participants and communities, which facilitate the conduct of essential health research. A concern with 'relational ethics', simply put, means thinking carefully about these relationships.

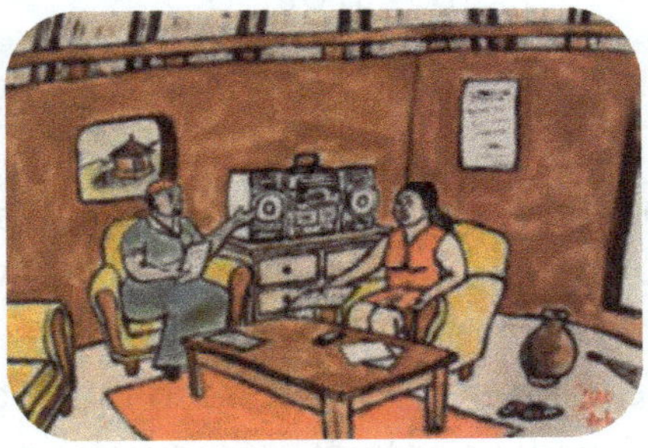

RESEARCH IS ABOUT RELATIONSHIPS

It also means thinking beyond and outside of the wealth of regulations which have sprung up in the field of transnational medical research. Relational ethics are the complex and spontaneous momentary pursuit of morally right actions in personal interactions with other humans. They are guided not so much by formal rules as by individual and social conscience, and by particular overlapping identities and relationships. Good clinical practice guidelines will tell you what you need to include in a participant information sheet for a research study. But they won't help you think through what to do, for example, if members of your team are labelled 'Satanists' by the community, if a participant says her child is hungry during a research appointment, or if one colleague makes a derogatory comment about another because of their gender, faith or ethnicity. Guidelines and regulations do not account for the 'messiness' of everyday encounters involved in global research practices.

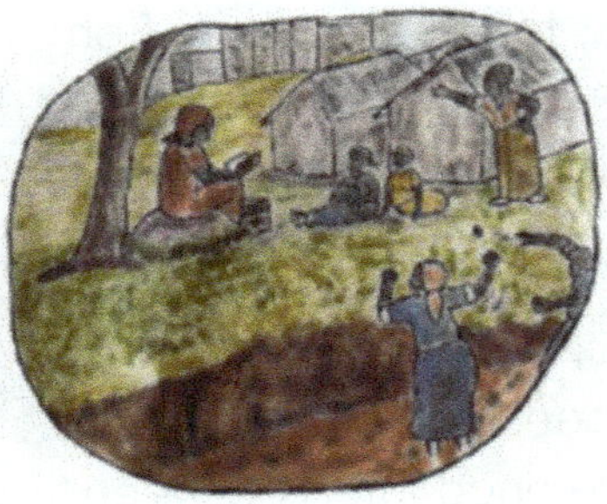

SATANISTS AT WORK

ANTHROPOLOGY AND RELATIONAL ETHICS

Anthropologists, on the other hand, have made the messiness of life their subject of enquiry. Anthropology is the study of human behaviour and human relationships. Anthropologists learn about this by spending long periods of time living in, and observing, different communities around the world. In our case, these were the communities of people involved in medical research in Africa.

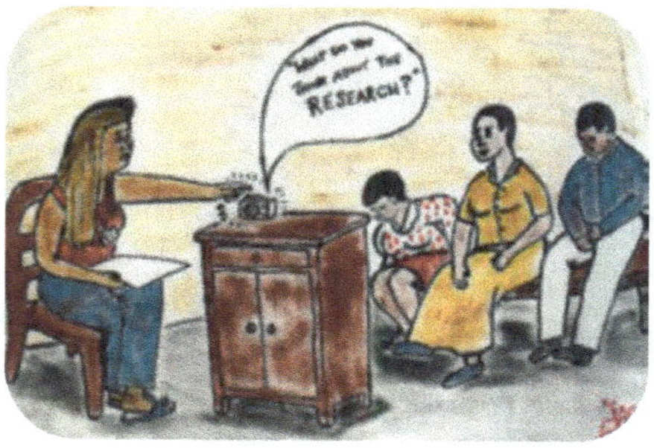

RESEARCHING RESEARCH

For the past decade we have been involved in, and conducted studies on, transnational medical research in different parts of Africa, in many cases at long-established, large-scale research sites. Our aim is to explore how medical research works in practice, and what ideas and hopes actors pursue through their work in their relations with others.

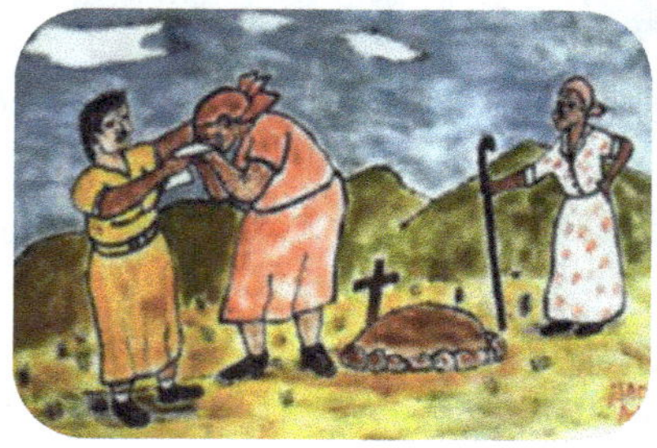

ANTHROPOLOGY: LEARNING BY BEING WITH PEOPLE THROUGH ALL ASPECTS OF THEIR LIVES

To collect data on 'relational ethics', we shadowed fieldworkers, sat in on senior staff meetings, and lived in the homes of research participants. We paid close attention to mundane practices and tacit knowledge, as well as hidden tensions, subtle cues, and complex moralities. We did this over long periods of time so that we could understand individual encounters and incidents in their wider contexts. At the same time, we also engaged ourselves in research collaborations, sought our informants' consent, underwent ethical review and faced ethical dilemmas – much in the same way as our colleagues in the medical sciences do. We tried to learn from the ethical reflections that arose from our own research too and, needless to say, we more often than not failed to achieve definite, satisfactory solutions to the challenges that, ultimately, stem from the unjust distribution of wealth between the world's peoples, as well as between academic and scholarly institutions.

During this process, we gathered many stories – some we were part of, others we followed as they unfolded, or were about told by colleagues. These stories have been fictionalized for the training case studies, but they are not hypothetical. They represent live encounters between researchers, participants and communities, and they show that ethics in medical research is complex and fluid, involving more than regulations and rules. Personal, cultural, professional, and community moralities and perspectives are all brought into play in specific contexts and situations.

RELATIONAL ETHICS AND INEQUALITY IN AFRICA

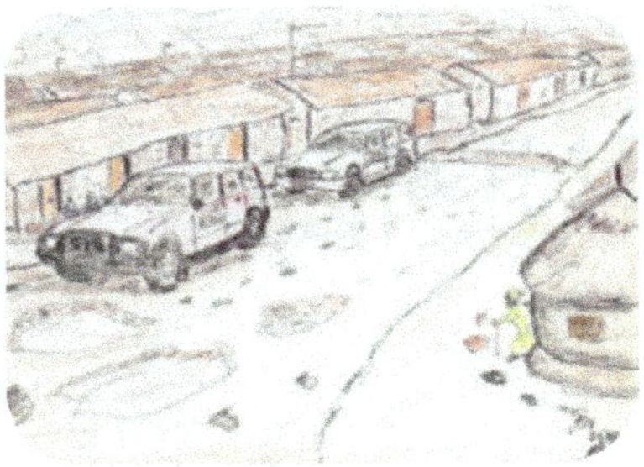

INEQUALITIES ARE SOMETIMES HIGHLY VISIBLE IN RESEARCH

Reflecting on relational ethics is important in any medical research context, but particularly crucial in Africa where global health research invariably involves major economic and political inequalities. The vast majority of health research conducted in Africa involves partnerships between countries, populations, institutions and staff from the global 'North' (the former European colonial powers and their North American successors), and their counterparts in the global 'South' (roughly speaking the formerly colonized areas of the globe). This means medical research in Africa operates across huge differentials in power, resources, and knowledge. Both the current reality of these differences, and historical memories of colonial relationships and post-colonial attempts at redress, affect how people involved in research today relate to each other. We found that these differences were an underlying theme to many of the ethical dilemmas we describe in this teaching resource. With this in mind we encourage both facilitators and training participants to read and engage with the material presented in the second half of this book which explores the current and historical context of transnational medical research and ethics in Africa in more depth.

Such things are often hard to talk about. Being explicit about inequality – and its many small practical effects – can be embarrassing, even humiliating. It can also highlight irresolvable differences in opinion, and therefore seem futile. This is why this workbook uses stories, rather than real cases. It is our hope that discussing the stories will give global health researchers the opportunity to think about how they manage dilemmas and uncomfortable research encounters across power divides.

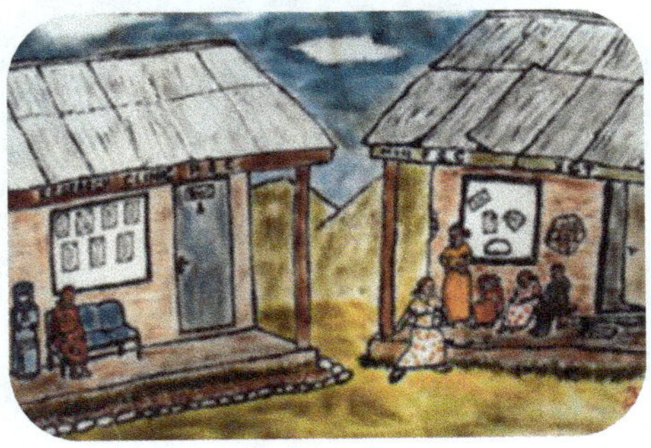

PATIENTS NOTICED THE SUBTLE DIFFERENCE BETWEEN THE GOVERNMENT CLINIC AND THE RESEARCH CLINIC

Our aim is to create a training tool which can begin to fill the gap between ethics guidelines and their implementation. The stories are designed to encourage practical thinking within constrained conditions, in order to improve the immediate conduct of medical research. But, at the same time we aim to raise awareness of the underlying, more challenging, issue of global inequality and how it affects global health research. The case studies are set up to encourage ethical deliberations on the stories to move between three distinct arenas of debate and action: debate over individual choices and behaviour, debate over institutional practices, and debate over wider 'structural' issues. An awareness of all three of these 'levels' operating in global medical research is, in our view, essential for all involved to move forward with a wider and more empowered understanding of ethical dilemmas.

PART ONE: TRAINING CASE STUDIES

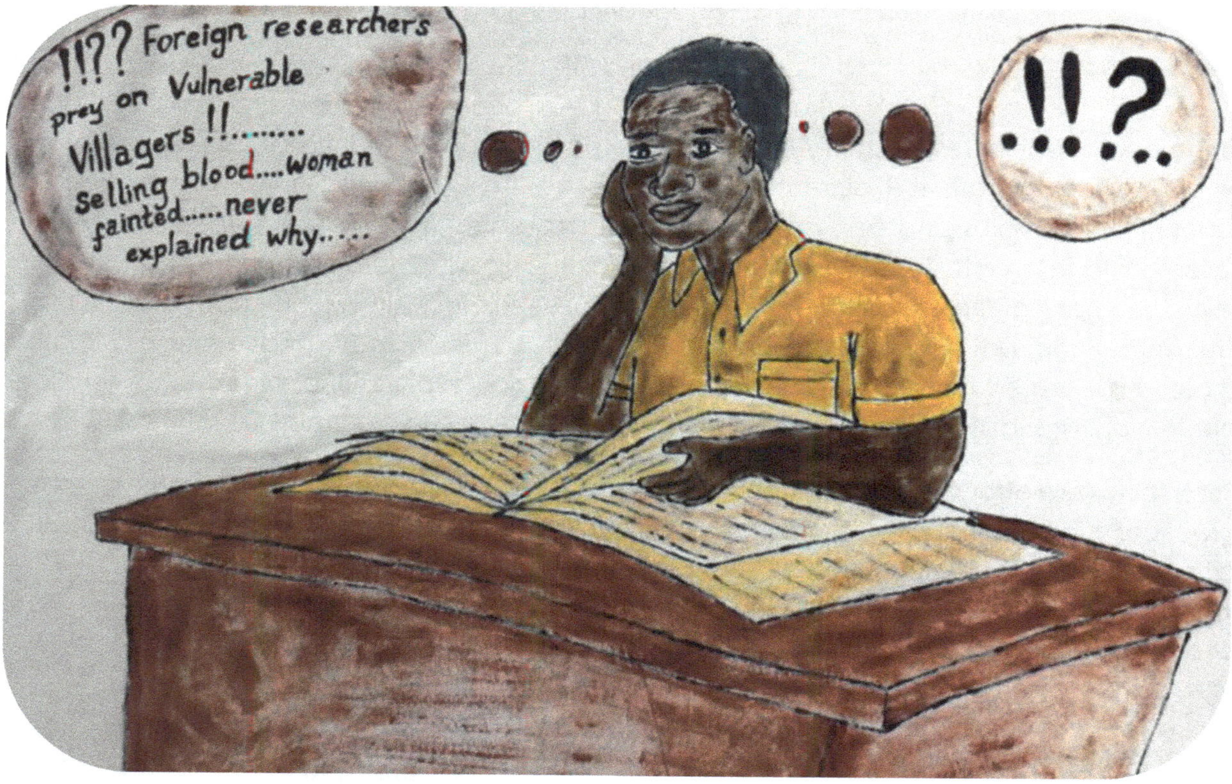
!!?? Foreign researchers prey on Vulnerable Villagers !!........ selling blood....woman fainted.....never explained why.....
.!!?..

'THINKING ABOUT THESE THINGS WAS NOT GOING TO BE EASY', THOUGHT ALOUIS.

RESEARCHER-PARTICIPANT RELATIONSHIPS

TRAINING CASE STUDIES

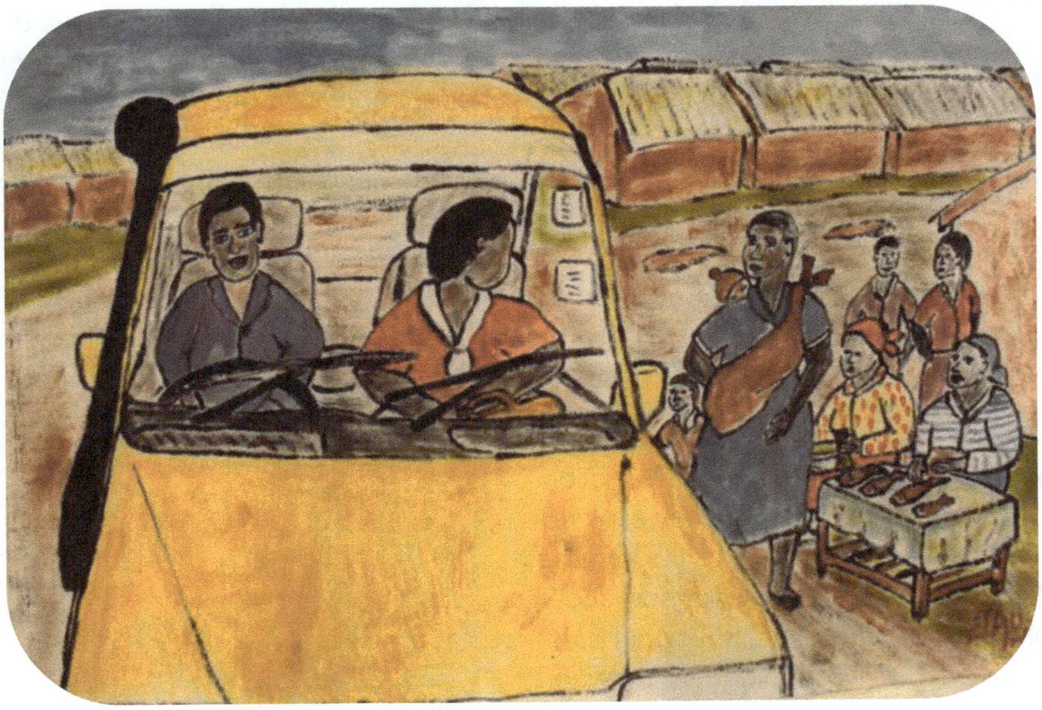

EVERYONE WAS WONDERING: WHO WAS CARO'S SMARTLY DRESSED 'FRIEND' WITH THE BIG CAR...?

RESEARCHER-PARTICIPANT RELATIONSHIPS
CASE STUDIES

How can we best categorize the relationship between researcher and participant? One is paid; the other is not, yet is not a customer or receiving a service. One seems more powerful, yet cannot function without the other; he or she cannot proceed in the relationship without the other's explicit consent. They are not friends, yet often share intimate details – albeit one-sided – about their lives. Their relationship is at once highly technical and sometimes deeply human. Furthermore, it is one which, while at first glance – in the moment of drawing blood or obtaining consent – seems to be a relationship between two individuals, in reality stands for relationships between whole populations, countries, governments and institutions.

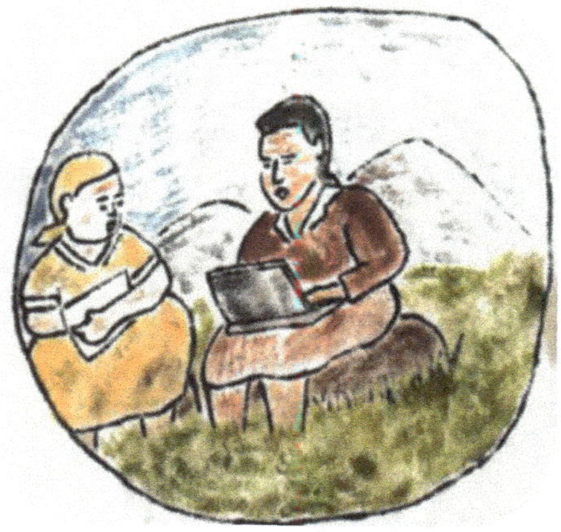

COLLECTING INFORMATION, CONNECTING WITH PEOPLE

The stories in this section concern this unique relationship. They explore standard ethical concerns such as the informed consent process, coercion, and transparency. They also explore less commonly talked about issues such as friendship and kin-like relationships between researchers and participants, as well as the emotional struggle researchers sometimes deal with when faced with the conditions of abject poverty experienced by some participants. The stories look at relational ethical dilemmas, such as when research clinicians faced with sick participants are forced to decide whether to be foremost researchers, or clinicians.

FURTHER READING

Special Issue: Fieldworkers at the interface between research institutions and local communities. *Developing World Bioethics* 13(1)

FIELDWORK AND FRIENDSHIP:
WORKING IN YOUR OWN COMMUNITY

FACILITATOR'S NOTES

This story focuses on the blurred lines between fieldwork and friendship when researchers are employed in their own communities.

Many research organizations rely heavily on the unique expertise of local community interviewers (also called 'villager reporters', 'community health workers', etc.), who are valued for their local understanding and their ability to negotiate both individual and collective consent. However, the personal position of such a worker is delicate, as they may feel pressure to represent the interests of both the research organization and the trial participants. Many conflicts and misunderstandings between organizations and their target communities are related to competition for limited employment in an already challenging economic environment. Paid interviewers often have to deal with resentment of their own economic good fortune, at the same time as working to encourage community members to participate in projects for free. Local staff may also be working directly with research participants who are friends or relatives, which adds extra pressure. How do they handle this?

This case study is designed both to encourage staff members in similar situations to express their personal challenges, and to help senior staff better understand these challenges. As such, care needs to be taken when setting the ground rules for this discussion. The facilitator needs to think carefully about the possible consequences of encouraging staff to open up about this topic. Many research organizations have strict rules governing conduct between researchers and participants. Will

LEARNING OBJECTIVE

To consider the challenges of working for research programmes in one's own community, especially when competing for limited employment opportunities, and to identify possible solutions

KEYWORDS

Informed consent

Community-based fieldworkers

Friendship

Employment issues

there be any consequences for staff if you encourage them to speak freely? The range of the discussion should be made clear at the beginning and this may involve extra preparation to create a 'safe space'. For example, if possible it would be helpful to be able to assure participants that there will be no disciplinary action if they discuss personal experiences that may have violated regulatory ethics. If this is not possible, we recommend you steer the discussion carefully away from areas where disclosure could lead to staff being disciplined later. The final discussion should include a discussion and comparison of different types of ethics – regulatory, and relational or individual.

FIELDWORK AND FRIENDSHIP:
WORKING IN YOUR OWN COMMUNITY

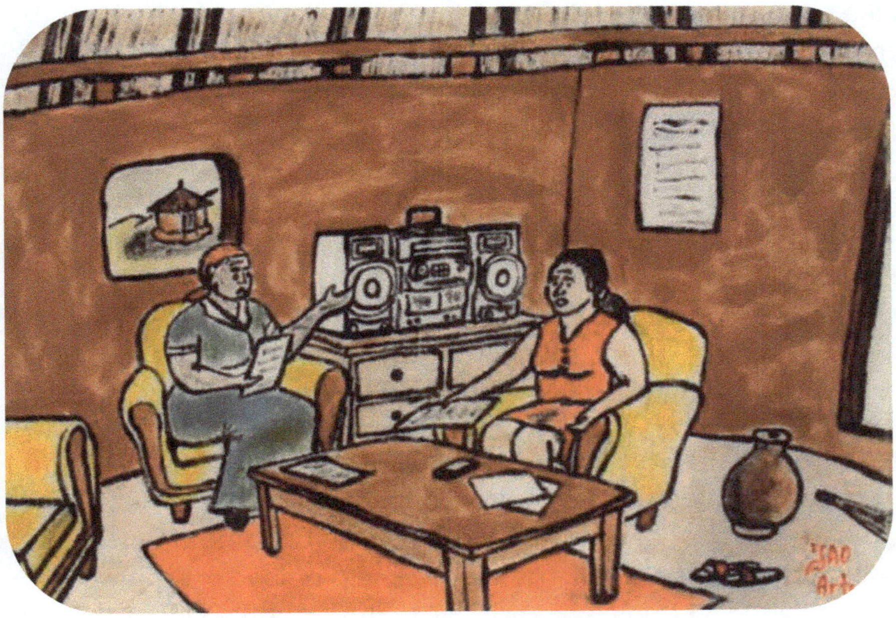

THE TENSION WAS PALPABLE AS JENNY READ MAGGIE THE CONSENT FORM

THE STORY

Jenny is a community interviewer for a transnational research organization, and is employed on a casual contract to work in her own marital village, where she has a long history of community work. As well as casual work for the research organization, she provides voluntary home-based care for people living with HIV/AIDS. She is also the secretary of a local network of women's self-help groups, and a church teacher. She has helped the research station on a number of projects over the past ten years, and has gone on numerous training courses.

At the moment, Jenny is working on a project looking at the feasibility of distributing condoms to women door-to-door. Her role is to visit women in their homes, explain the study to them and obtain their informed consent. Today she visits Maggie, a younger woman living with her husband and child. Maggie is a teacher working in a nearby school so Jenny visits her on the weekend when she knows she will be in. Jenny and Maggie have known each other for a long time. Before Maggie trained to be a teacher, Jenny organized for her to assist her as a village reporter on a research project. But, after that project finished, Maggie was not asked to assist again. Jenny says that this was because Maggie 'didn't know the right way to talk to people'.

When Jenny arrives at Maggie's home she is greeted cordially and invited to sit. After exchanging greetings and some local news, Jenny starts to explain the new study to Maggie. Soon, however, the atmosphere becomes a little awkward. Jenny stumbles over her words when reading the form and Maggie corrects her disdainfully. Maggie's husband arrives when they are still going through the consent form, and stays to listen. When they get to the end, Jenny asks Maggie if she is happy to be visited and given the condoms every month. Maggie says loudly, 'No, I do not consent. It is my right. Look here, it says I can say no. You need to say that it is my right to say no. Say that first.'

Jenny is a bit taken aback at Maggie's tone, but agrees that of course Maggie can say no. She looks for her pen. 'Look,' says Maggie, 'this lady is not prepared, where is her pen?' Maggie's husband is clearly uncomfortable. He asks Jenny to tell him what the research is about. But before Jenny can answer, Maggie tells him, 'Why are you asking her? I know what it is about.' Maggie and her husband start to bicker, and now Jenny is uncomfortable. She tells Maggie she will come back later for the consent form and leaves quickly.

Walking away, Jenny is clearly upset. A researcher accompanying her on the visit asks her what went wrong. 'I don't know,' replies Jenny, 'we used to be such good friends, and now look at the way she talks to me. She has become so arrogant since she became a teacher. I won't be able to do good work in that home again. Last month, she promised me she would take her child to the clinic for that vaccine study. She kept saying she was going to and then she didn't. In the end I arranged for a motorbike to take them. Then she left me to pay for it!'

'Do you think it was because I was there?' the researcher asks. 'Perhaps,' Jenny replies. 'I don't know. I think she is also having some problems with her husband. He has been staying away a lot. I did hear he might be getting a second wife.'

QUESTIONS

- There might be several reasons for the awkwardness that has developed between Jenny and Maggie. What might these be?
- Do you think Jenny's employers should know about what has happened? Why (or why not) might it matter to them?
- What should Jenny do, if anything?
- What should the research organization do, if anything?

GROUP ACTIVITY

Divide into two groups. Drawing on their own experience, the first group brainstorms the ethical dilemmas and possible tensions somebody like Jenny may face. Again drawing on their own experience, the second group explores the benefits of working within your own community, like Jenny does. Are there situations where fieldworkers can actually avoid ethical challenges, or act more ethically, because of their unique position and knowledge of their own community?

Then the two groups present their points to each other. Do the benefits outweigh the challenges?

FURTHER READING

Chantler, T., Otewa, F. et al. (2013) Ethical challenges that arise at the community interface of health research: village reporters' experiences in Western Kenya. *Developing World Bioethics* 13(1), 30–37.

Kamuya, D.M., Theobald, S.J. et al. (2013) Evolving friendships and shifting ethical dilemmas: fieldworkers' experiences in a short term community based study in Kenya. *Developing World Bioethics* 13(1), 1–9.

Simon, C. and Mosavel, M. (2010) Community members as recruiters of human subjects: ethical considerations. *American Journal of Bioethics* 10(3), 3–11.

SOAP AND PERSUASION:

RECRUITING AND CARING FOR PARTICIPANTS

FACILITATOR'S NOTES

This case study is about the way a study recruiter relates to and interacts with potential participants, and raises the question of whether his interactions are ethical. It is a useful scenario to use to encourage discussion about the challenges fieldworkers encounter, and how these can be managed ethically. The case study prompts broader questions about benefits, inducements, coercion, and the distinction between research activities and meeting participants' basic public health needs. In this story a government public health worker is seconded to a research project, raising issues around different work experiences and goals. This case study can, therefore, also be used to make connections to themes arising in the Institutional Relationships group of case studies.

You may not be able to cover all of this ground in your session, so in directing the discussion, it may be useful to think about who your training participants are, what questions engage them most in their work, and what changes they may be in a position to make. This does not mean that you should not touch upon all these questions, but you may want to decide on what you will focus on in most depth.

LEARNING OBJECTIVE

To recognise that the balance between professional involvement and personal relationships is both a practical and a moral challenge for staff who interact directly with research participants, and to consider various possible views of the role of medical research in communities

KEYWORDS

Informed consent

Inducements

Government

Poverty

SOAP AND PERSUASION:
RECRUITING AND CARING FOR PARTICIPANTS

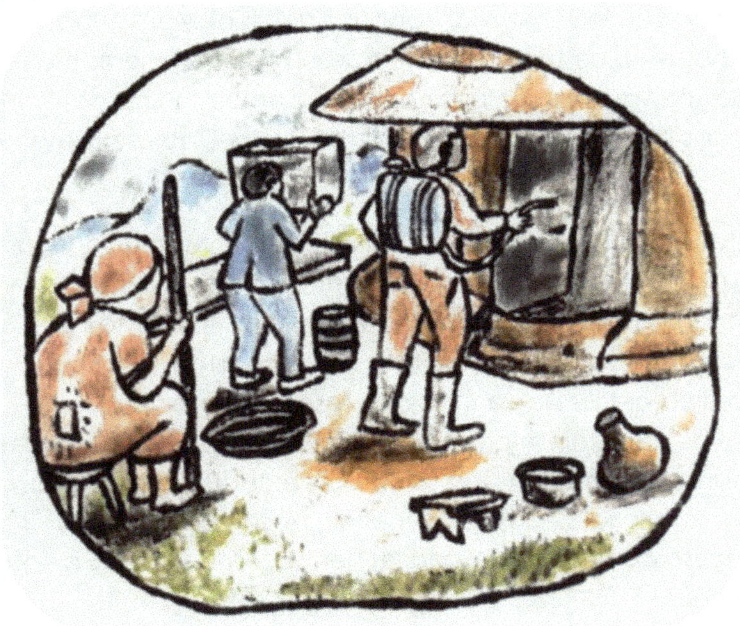

MAMA JANE WATCHED AS THE RESEARCHERS REMOVED ALL HER THINGS

THE STORY

A research study looking at the cost-effectiveness of indoor residual house spraying (IRS) is taking place in Malawi. The study is being carried out by a Danish university in collaboration with a Malawian research institute. The study involves spraying 1,000 houses over a few days, every six months. The researchers have asked local government public health officials for assistance with this, so four public health officials are seconded to the study on a temporary basis to help with the spraying, and with obtaining consent from the household heads.

David, one of these public health officials, has a huge amount of experience in community public health work. He is highly respected, and known locally as 'Pastor-Doctor' because he also preaches in one of the nearby Pentecostal churches. He is close to retirement age; several of the local researchers on the study received their first training in public health work from him, before getting jobs in more lucrative international research.

Soon it is time for the third and final round of spraying, and the study is going well. Relations with the community are good and consent rates are high, particularly among the homes visited by the public health officials, who are seen as 'community experts' by the researchers. For this last round, David is unable to visit one of the houses he has visited before so a local female researcher, Bilah, goes instead.

There have never been any reported problems with spraying this home, which belongs to an elderly widow known as Mama Jane. However, this time Bilah reports back that Mama Jane has refused to give her consent for her house to be sprayed. 'She doesn't like the research,' she tells the study coordinator. 'She doesn't want me moving her things outside the house where people can see them. And she says she wants the soap that the Pastor-Doctor always brings before he sprays her house.

David is called in for a meeting. The study coordinator accuses him of 'bribing' Mama Jane to take part, saying that his actions have invalidated the informed consent process. David is really angry. 'How can I "bribe" my grandmother?' he retorts. 'This widow has no one to take care of her. Did you not see the way her house was? How her things were so dirty? If I don't give her soap, who will?' The study coordinator tells David that, as a researcher, this isn't his concern. His role in this case should only be to obtain informed consent before spraying, which means that Mama Jane has to understand the research and freely agree. 'Ha!' replies David. 'What does that mean? She believes that malaria is caused by the rain. Are you telling me that because of this we should let her house go unsprayed, and let her become sick? IRS is not only about research. It's about public health!'

The study coordinator and David reach an impasse. David threatens to pull out of the study. The study coordinator is concerned about the effect this will have on community relations. He is also concerned about just how much soap has been circulating in the study area.

QUESTIONS

- What do you think are the key issues in this story?
- What do you think about researchers asking public health professionals to undertake recruitment for them? What are the consequences of this for recruitment practice?
- What do you think David means when he says 'How can I "bribe" my grandmother?' What other 'kinship' relationships seem to be at play among David, the researchers, the coordinator, and the community?
- What could be the consequences for the project if David leaves the study?
- Do you think that participants in this study should receive some form of reimbursement? If no, why not, and if yes, what should this be?
- What do you think about David's commentary on the public health aspect of the IRS? Do you agree? What challenges – and benefits – does this idea pose for researchers?

FURTHER READING

Chantler, T., Otewa, F. et al. (2013) Ethical challenges that arise at the community interface of health research: village reporters' experiences in Western Kenya. *Developing World Bioethics* 13(1), 30–37.

Geissler, P.W., Kelly, A., Imoukhuede B., Pool, R. (2008) 'He is now like a brother, I can even give him some blood' – relational ethics and material exchanges in a malaria vaccine 'trial community' in The Gambia. *Social Science and Medicine* 67(5), 696–707.

GEL AND/OR CONDOMS:

SAFETY IN A MICROBICIDE TRIAL

FACILITATOR'S NOTES

This story is about participants' understanding of the risks involved in research. It focuses on a woman taking part in a microbicide trial who appears to have understood the study information, but still chooses to use the gel in a way which puts her at risk of HIV infection. The aim of this case study is to encourage deeper reflection on how we interpret participants' understanding of the information we provide, and the extent of our responsibility to reduce the risks participants are exposed to – especially when they could be seen as 'vulnerable' in some way.

When thinking about informed consent and participants' understanding of risks, this study invites us to look beyond asking simply whether participants understand the basic facts. It is clear that the woman in this story understands the information she is given. However, despite the advice of the researchers, she takes a calculated risk, based partly on economic necessity and partly on her understanding of the context of the project. The question is whether she is more at risk of catching HIV as a result of taking part in the research, and, if so, what the responsibility – and ability – of the researchers might be to address this.

LEARNING OBJECTIVE

To move beyond a simplistic understanding of informed consent (in terms of simple comprehension of facts), and to reflect on the extent of researchers' responsibility towards reducing risks for vulnerable participants

KEYWORDS

Informed consent

Safety

Understanding risk

GEL AND/OR CONDOMS:

SAFETY IN A MICROBICIDE TRIAL

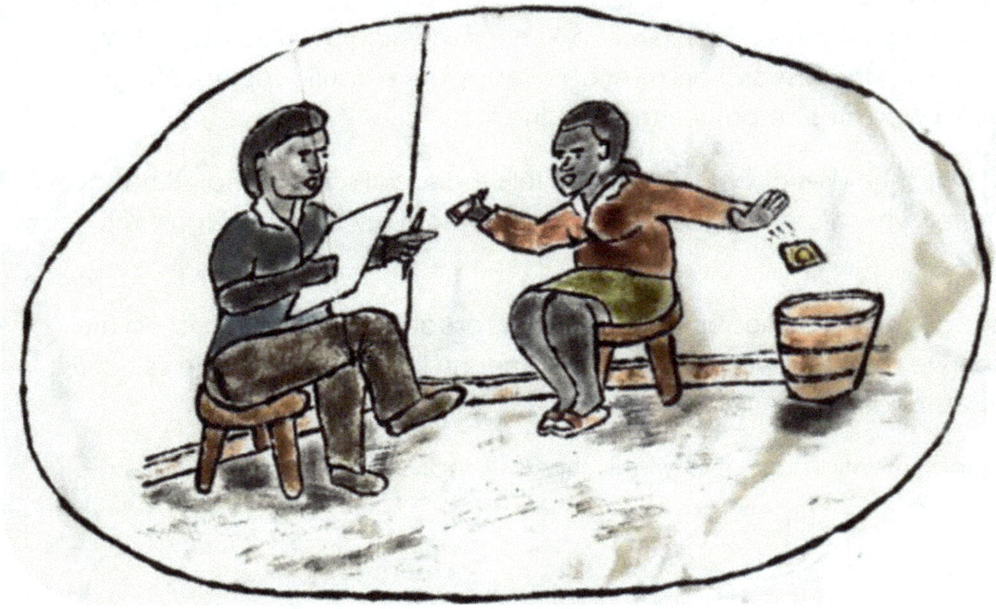

'EXCELLENT!' SAID LUCY, 'NOW I CAN THROW AWAY THESE CONDOMS'

THE STORY

Lucy is taking part in a trial to see if using a microbicide gel protects women in occupations with a high risk of HIV infection. Lucy is widowed and runs a makeshift bar behind her house. She brews local alcohol which she serves to a mainly male clientele. She does not consider herself a commercial sex worker, but sometimes for a little extra tip or a gift she does have sex with a few of her regular customers.

Lucy has been given information about the trial and the gel on a number of occasions: when the researchers first visited her bar to tell her about the trial; at a second visit to enroll her formally into the study; and every month when she comes to the research clinic for a study visit. Each time she is told that 'because we don't yet know whether the gel works, you must still use a condom. Proper use of a condom is the most effective form of HIV prevention.' Each time, Lucy is given the same information sheet to read, accompanied by a cartoon about the trial. And each time she is asked a series of questions by the staff to check she has understood the message. Lucy passes this test every time.

However, towards the end of the study a social scientist comes to do some in-depth interviews with some of the women about their experiences of the trial. Lucy is selected to participate. In her interview she tells the social scientist that she understands that the gel may not work, or that she may be using a placebo gel. She tells her that '"placebo" means fake'. But, she also tells the social scientist that she has been trying out the gel without using a condom because she wants 'to see if it works'. When the social scientist probes a bit deeper to understand what Lucy means, she says 'Well, if I use a condom, how will I know if the gel works? It will be the condom working, not the gel!' The social scientist asks her if she is not worried about HIV infection. Lucy tells her that the researchers must be already quite confident that the gel worked, otherwise they wouldn't be bothering to do the trial.

When Lucy is asked what she likes about the gel, she tells the social scientist that 'It has been helpful for me, because when I use the gel instead of a condom my boyfriends give me something extra.'

The social scientists report their findings back to the study researchers. The researchers are frustrated. 'What can we do,' they wonder, 'to stop someone like Lucy putting herself at risk? We thought she understood.'

'Well,' says the Principal Investigator, 'at least this shows us that effective microbicides are really needed.'

QUESTIONS

- What are key ethical issues at stake in this situation?
- Do you understand Lucy's decision?
- What do you think is the extent of researchers' responsibility to reduce the risk of HIV infection when offering participants an experimental HIV prevention tool? How could researchers assess their own efforts at this?
- Has participation in the study increased Lucy's risk of contracting HIV or other sexually transmitted infections?
- Is there anything else the study team could do to help Lucy use condoms? Is this their job?
- What do you make of the Principal Investigator's response?

REFLECTIONS ON YOUR OWN EXPERIENCE

Can you think of similar situations from your experience? How did you ensure participants were at minimal risk of harm? Did things ever work out unexpectedly, despite your best efforts? Looking back now, what might you have done differently?

ACTIVITIES

1. Split up into two groups, and devise an information sheet or activity to explain the importance of condom use for each sex act in a study similar to the one described above. Then, take in turns to use your information sheet/activity to inform the other group about your project. What potential issues that affect safety are not covered by the information? What situations can the group being informed imagine where they would not follow the advice being given? How can you best talk through these issues with the participants?
2. In 2013, the Vaginal and Oral Interventions to Control the Epidemic (Voice) trial, a multi-sited study in South Africa, Ugandan and Zimbabwean hit the global news headlines when researchers revealed that blood tests showed that many participants had lied about their adherence to the products being tested. The study aimed to test whether a daily anti-retroviral pill or once-a-day vaginal gel would protect at-risk women from contracting HIV. The women were blamed in the global press for deliberate deception and for participating in the research only for "stipends". This led to a debate about the morality of clinical trials. A group of anthropologists conducted some interviews with the South African participants to explore the meaning of the lie from the perspectives of the women themselves. Read a summary of their findings here: https://theconversation.com/what-drove-women-to-lie-in-an-hiv-clinical-trial-in-southern-africa-51143 and discuss the implications in your group for designing future trials. In what way is what happened in the VOICE study different to Lucy's story above? In what way is it similar?

FURTHER READING

Beskow, L.M. and McCall, J. (Eds). *Informed Consent. Rethinking clinical trials: a living textbook of pragmatic clinical trials.* NIH Health Care Systems Research Collaboratory. Available at: http://sites.duke.edu/rethinkingclinicaltrials/informed-consent-in-pragmatic-clinical-trials (accessed 25 October 2015).

Corneli, A.L. et al. (2012) Improving participant understanding of informed consent in an HIV-prevention clinical trial: a comparison of methods. *Aids and Behaviour* 16(2), 412–421.

Cooper, M. (2013) Double exposure – sex workers, biomedical prevention trials, and the dual logic of global public health. *S & F Online* 11(3), 1–11.

Kingori, P. (2015) When the science fails and the ethics works: 'Fail-safe' ethics in the FEM-PrEP study. *Anthropology and Medicine* Epub 2015 Oct 20, 1-17

Moodley, K. (2007) Microbicide research in developing countries: have we given the ethical concerns due consideration? *BMC Medical Ethics* 2007 Sep 19, 8:10.

Mystakidou, K. et al. (2009) Ethical and practical challenges in implementing informed consent in HIV/AIDS clinical trials in developing or resource-limited countries. *SAHARA J* 6(2), 46–57.

Stadler, J., et al. (2015) Adherence and the Lie in a HIV Prevention Clinical Trial. *Medical Anthropology:* 1-14.

Vallely, A. et al. (2010) How informed is consent in vulnerable populations? Experience using a continuous consent process during the MDP301 vaginal microbicide trial in Mwanza, Tanzania. *BMC Medical Ethics* 2010 Jun 13, 11:10.

FRIENDS LIKE HOW?: GETTING PERSONALLY INVOLVED WITH PARTICIPANTS

FACILITATOR'S NOTES

The story in this case study is about a friendship that develops between an expatriate social researcher and a research participant. It deals with questions of boundaries in research relationships, and with confidentiality and trust. The different backgrounds of the two individuals in this relationship are striking, but similar situations can occur with local researchers and study participants. You might want to point this out in your discussions, and talk about whether this raises similar or different challenges.

The question of friendship and ongoing connections can become particularly important at the end of a study, when research staff have to tell participants that they will no longer be visiting them or seeing them at clinic. In situations where participants are in evident need, or are socially isolated, this can be very difficult, and some staff might choose to remain in contact with certain participants. It would be good to think about the consequences of this, and also to consider the role of culture, and the fact that some participants might live in the same neighbourhood as research staff.

The other key theme this case study touches on is confidentiality, both in terms of disclosing how the two people meet, and how the relationship helps the researcher collect 'rich' data for the study. How should the researcher manage this ethically? Should she leave her friend out of her write-up of the research, or just try to ensure she understands that some of her experiences will be included in the research? These are important questions which need to be considered carefully, bearing in mind that different research disciplines use different approaches to data collection

LEARNING OBJECTIVE

To explore personal closeness and boundaries in research relationships, especially at the end of trials

KEYWORDS

Confidentiality

Friendship

FRIENDS LIKE HOW?:

GETTING PERSONALLY INVOLVED WITH PARTICIPANTS

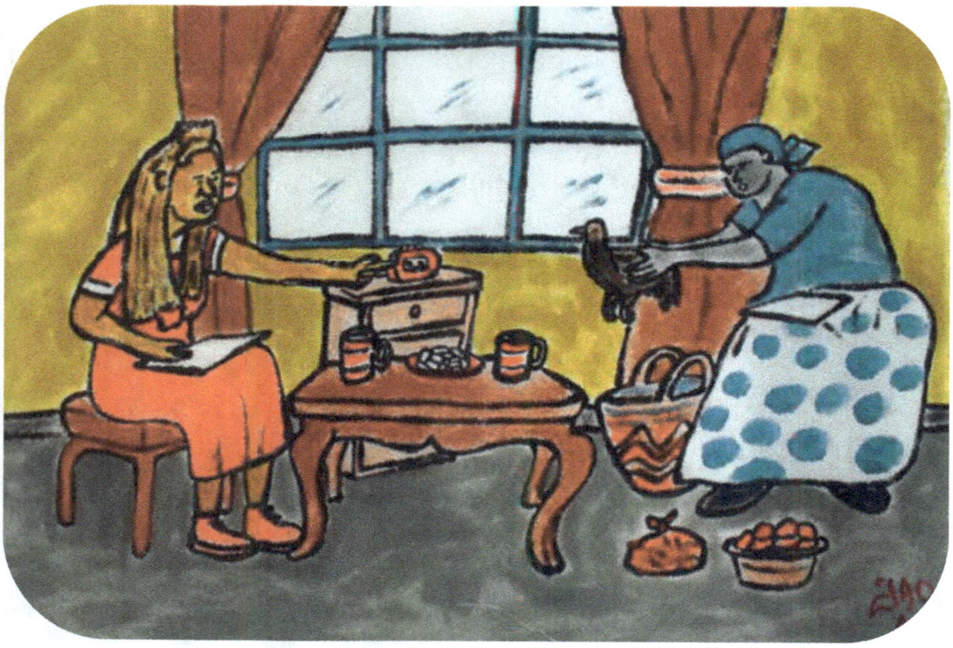

AS JANE SWITCHED ON THE RECORDER, SALLY HANDED HER A CHICKEN.

THE STORY

Jane, an overseas social scientist, is attached to a clinical study of HIV positive men and women taking place in an African city. As part of her research she conducts in-depth interviews with some participants and accompanies them on clinic visits. One of these participants is Sally. Jane spends a long time interviewing Sally in Jane's own home, as there is nowhere else Sally feels comfortable talking about her HIV status. During their second interview Sally asks Jane if they could 'become friends'. Jane is a little cautious about being asked such a direct question; she wants to know exactly what Sally means, and asks, 'Friends like how?' Sally replies, 'Friends who talk to each other.' In their next few interviews Sally shares a lot with Jane. She tells her about the difficulties she has with her husband, who refuses to talk about his own HIV status and will not go for a test.

A few weeks later, Jane hears that Sally's CD4 count has dropped and she needs to start treatment. Jane knows that this will be upsetting for Sally, because she has talked a lot about the fact she was proud she was not on treatment. Jane knows it will be a shock. She also knows from her interviews with Sally that Sally reacts to shock with initial silence. In one of the clinical study meetings, Jane hears the staff saying that they are worried that Sally will not come to the clinic for the treatment 'because of stigma from her husband' and that it is quite an urgent situation. Jane does not know what to do. She feels sure that Sally intends to participate, but is just taking a day to recover from the shock. She considers calling Sally to encourage her, but feels she should not repeat what she has heard about Sally in the clinical study meeting. She also feels that she cannot tell the clinical study staff about what she knows about Sally's character from the in-depth interviews, as this would be breaking Sally's confidentiality. So she waits a few days, all the time quite worried about Sally.

Then Sally herself sends Jane a text message. She just says she has had a big shock and is feeling lost. She does not give any more details. She asks Jane if she would be able to accompany her to the clinic 'as a friend'. Jane agrees. Jane and Sally arrive early at the clinic. Jane brings a thermos of tea which they share while Sally talks about what has happened. When she found out she needed to start treatment, she told her husband, who already knew her status, but he just walked away and has said nothing more about the issue since then. She says she called Jane because she needed 'moral support' to attend the clinic.

Sally asks Jane to come in to see the doctor with her. Jane thinks about reminding Sally that she is also a researcher, and so would be observing with 'two hats on', but it does not feel like this is the right moment. Instead, she quickly makes sure that the doctor is happy for her to accompany Sally.

The doctor talks to both Jane and Sally, saying they should speak in English for Jane. Jane finds herself thinking 'English would be better for my research!' But then mentally rebukes herself, and tells them to use whichever language they prefer. She pretends she can understand the local language better than she actually can, and wishes she had a tape-recorder to translate later. Jane also accompanies Sally to have her blood taken and to see the pharmacist. Because of the language issue, Jane isn't entirely clear what happens in all these sessions.

Afterwards, Sally tells Jane that she cannot imagine how she could have even entered the clinic alone, as she was still in shock. For the rest of the study, which is nearing its end, the study staff refer to Sally as 'Jane's friend'. Sometimes they tell Jane things about Sally and her treatment that Sally herself does not discuss with her. Jane feels very awkward about this and does not want to get caught in the middle. While staff praise her for supporting Sally, Jane feels conflicted because although her main motivation is to be helpful, she has also gathered a lot of data for her research from the experience. She is still not clear if Sally understands this aspect of their relationship.

After the study ends, Sally takes courage and goes to register at the HIV Care and Support Centre by herself. Several years later, Jane and Sally are still very good friends; they have met each other's families, slept in each other's houses, and attended funerals and weddings together. Sally is very private about her HIV status. She tells people who ask how she knows Jane that they met as 'pen-friends'. But she doesn't tell Jane this, so when asked by Sally's father-in-law, Jane says 'we met just around on the streets'.

QUESTIONS

- How would you describe what happened here? What are the key ethical issues?
- Why do you think Jane was initially cautious when Sally asked to be friends?
- Why do you think Sally called Jane in particular to go with her to the clinic?
- Do you think Jane did the right thing? For whom? Could she have done some things differently? Do you think there could have been any problematic consequences from this situation? For whom? Sally? Jane? The clinical study?
- Do you think this was a one-off unique situation for either Jane or Sally?
- Do you think Jane's research suffered or benefited from what happened?
- What part do 'rapport' and 'relationships' play in your own work?

REFLECTION ON YOUR OWN EXPERIENCE

Can you think of any similar situations from your experience? How did you deal with them? Looking back now, what could you have done differently?

ACTIVITY

Split into small groups and think about the nature of relationships in social research, and how to manage the boundaries between friendship and acquaintance. List the advantages and disadvantages of Jane's agreeing to befriend Sally, and think about what might have happened if she had explained that she could not be her friend due to her relationship with her as a researcher. Discuss and then vote on whether Jane should describe in her research what she has learned from her relationship with Sally.

FURTHER READING

Madiega, P.A., Jones, G. et al. (2013). 'She's my sister-In-law, my visitor, my friend' – challenges of staff identity in home follow-up in an HIV trial in Western Kenya. *Developing World Bioethics* 13(1), 21–29

READABILITY AND SWEET TALK:

TRANSLATION AND COMPREHENSION OF STUDY DOCUMENTS

FACILITATOR'S NOTES

This case study is about the translation and comprehension of study information, and it also raises questions about how such information should be delivered – for example, during the consent process should fieldworkers be able to use their own words to illustrate particular points? This story could be useful during the run-up to a new project, when study documents are being prepared and decisions are being made about recruiting participants.

There are two main areas for discussion here: the first is about the translation process, and the second is about how information is exchanged between research staff and participants. It would be good to think carefully about what is meant by 'sweetening' the words on the consent form, and how this might be different from using colloquial terms to illustrate certain points. Questions of trust and protocol between the Principal Investigator and the staff also emerge.

LEARNING OBJECTIVE

To think more widely about the translation of study documents, considering local variations in language, the different ways participants interpret terms and facts, and the role of social relations in the information process

KEYWORDS

Informed consent

Translation

Comprehension

Documents

READABILITY AND SWEET TALK:

TRANSLATION AND COMPREHENSION OF STUDY DOCUMENTS

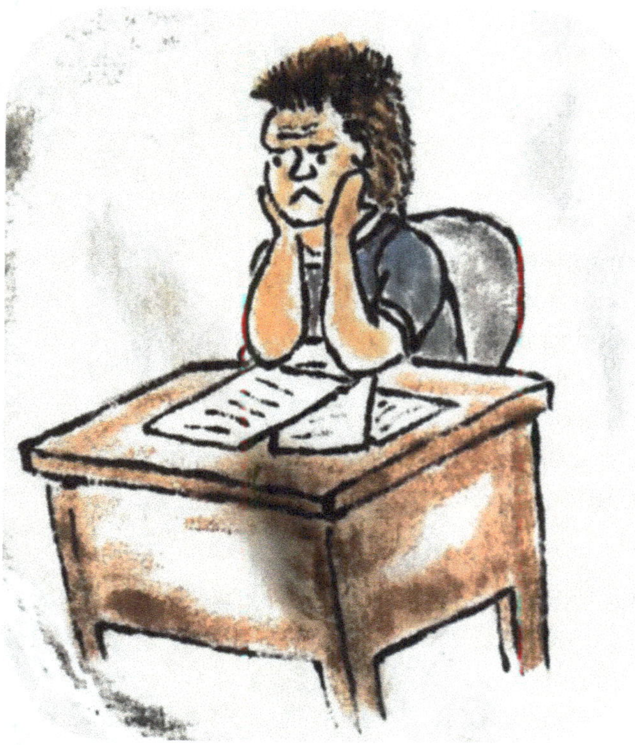

THE P.I LOOKED AT THE TRANSLATED CONSENT FORMS IN DESPAIR

THE STORY

The Institutional Review Board in this African country requires consent forms to be rated for their 'readability' using the Flesch-Kincaid grading system. The Flesch-Kincaid system uses word and sentence length to assess readability. After achieving an appropriate rating, the English forms are translated and back-translated to and from local languages, by staff who consider themselves fluent. This country has a large number of tribes, each with their own 'mother-tongue'. The linguistic situation is complicated further by the existence of local sub-tribes and clans, who speak variants of the tribal languages.

Despite achieving high readability scores in her consent forms in English, the British Principal Investigator of a TB study encounters endless problems when they are translated. She initially asks two native speakers to do separate translations: the study coordinator, who grew up in a city, and a younger fieldworker who grew up in the rural area where the study will take place. The translations they produce look quite different. Despite speaking the same local language, they disagree about certain words, as well as how to translate English words for which there is no straightforward equivalent. After some discussion, several other staff members are drafted in to help, and a working consensus is reached. The final translated consent form contains some English words, and is considerably longer than the English original. The Principal Investigator worries whether it will still have an acceptable 'readability' grade if the Flesch-Kincaid formula were applied, but as there is no equivalent system for testing readability in the local languages, she decides to proceed.

However, when the consent forms are used in the field she discovers that her problems are not over. The forms are used by fieldworkers who are, mostly, one or more generations older than the staff who translated the forms. They were instructed to read the forms aloud to participants, but in practice some of them stumble over the words, and the participants do not always appear to be reading along with them. The fieldworkers often follow the text with their fingers, and seem to repeat many of the sentences again after getting to the end of them. It seems to take a long, awkward time for the fieldworkers to read out the form, and the participants usually do not have any questions about the study at the end. This suggests that they have not really understood.

Sometimes, however, the fieldworker would abandon the form after a short time and talk casually about the study with the participant. The participants seem to ask more questions in these cases. The fieldworkers' off-the-cuff descriptions of the study seem to be different from the formal written descriptions. For example, fieldworkers are asked to say they are looking for pregnant women to include in a sub-study. But instead, they tend to say that they would be looking out for 'any women whose skin had become very beautiful and smooth recently'.

When asked about their experiences using the form, the fieldworkers say that the forms were good and made sense. But when they are probed a bit further, it emerges that both the fieldworkers and participants are not used to reading in their local language. Those that can read and write tend to do so in English. The Principal Investigator asks if it would be better to use forms written in English. 'No,' the fieldworkers reply, 'most participants do not really understand English.'

'What about making the sentences shorter?' she asks. 'Would that help?' 'Well,' they reply, 'mother-tongue is different from English; the meaning is not in the sentences but in the whole thing. You have to get to the end to know what the beginning means.'

Despite the difficulties with reading the form aloud, the Principal Investigator cautions the fieldworkers against abandoning the form and using their own words to describe the study. 'It is important that all the participants hear the same messages,' she says. 'When they sign that form, they are signing to say that they have heard all of it.' The fieldworkers reply: 'But sometimes we need to sweeten the words of the form. Otherwise people will say we are disrespectful. You can't say some of it just like that. You need to take the participants slowly.'

'So what should we do?' wonders the Principal Investigator.

QUESTIONS

- How would you measure the Flesch-Kincaid grade of this case study?
- What do you think grading systems can measure? What can't they measure?
- Is the readability of a form the same as participants being able to comprehend a study?
- There are several different issues about the use of consent forms signposted here. Can you disentangle and list them?
- The study coordinator and the young fieldworker produce different translations of the form. Can you think of several reasons why?
- Why does the finalized translation not always work in the field?
- Why do you think the fieldworkers don't ask directly about pregnancy?
- What do you think the older fieldworkers meant by 'sweetening' the words of the form?
- What does this case tell you about the nature of language? Can you think of different ways you use one language, in different contexts?
- How do you think the Principal Investigator feels, about her relationship with her staff and the ethics of the study? If you were her, what would you do next?
- Are there alternative ways of getting informed consent to using written forms?

ACTIVITY

Divide into groups, and, if you are in a group where people speak several languages, try to translate the following paragraph and compare notes. Where do you find differences or challenges? Even if you do not speak any other languages, do you think any parts may be problematic? What solutions can you come up with?

> *We invite you to take part in a study. The study is conducted by EMRC/HTW. This study is investigating the current prevalence of TB among the general population in your area. We also want to know the prevalence of TB among pregnant women. As part of this*

study fieldworkers will be visiting people in their homes and collecting sputum samples from all willing household members over the age of 18. The fieldworkers will also offer female participants over the age of 18 pregnancy tests. The information below will help you decide whether you are happy to participate in the study.

FURTHER READING

Kithinji, C. and Kass, N.E. (2010) Assessing the readability of non-English-language consent forms: the case of Kiswahili for research conducted in Kenya. *IRB: Ethics & Human Research* 32 (4), 10–15.

Mack, N., Ramirez, C.B., Friedland, B., and Nnko, S. (2013) Lost in translation: assessing effectiveness of focus group questioning techniques to develop improved translation of terminology used in HIV prevention clinical trials. *PLoS One* 8(9): e73799.

WE DON'T PAY:
'BUS FARES' AND OTHER GIFTS IN RESEARCH

FACILITATOR'S NOTES

Research participants usually receive reimbursement for their transport costs to research clinics. Often this is provided as a fixed amount rather than on provision of a receipt. From the perspective of research protocols, transport reimbursement is just that – reimbursement for transport. But it might have a different meaning for research participants. This story asks why, and whether it matters.

The story describes a woman participating in a diabetes care study, who despite being in poor health wants to walk to the clinic in order to keep her transport money. This poses a challenge to the research staff, who feel responsible for participant welfare as well as abiding to standard operating procedures.

Invite your group to think about practical solutions to this dilemma. However, you could also extend the discussion to reflect on how you think research participants really view their involvement. It is clear that the research participant in this story sees the transport reimbursement as a direct benefit of participation. Normally she receives it as fixed amount which is the same as all other participants, regardless of where they live in relation to the clinic or how they travel there. She may have come to depend on this money for expenses like food. This time, however, her worsening condition means that the research team bring her to the clinic. Suddenly the transport reimbursement she has previously viewed as a direct cash benefit becomes money that has to be explicitly used for transport.

For research participants living in challenging social and economic conditions, the relatively small amounts offered as

LEARNING OBJECTIVE

To reflect on the meaning and value of monetary payments in research among poor populations

KEYWORDS

Money

Poverty

Inducements

Informed consent

Personal morality

transport reimbursement are comparable to daily wages obtained through casual labour. Does this mean it equates to payment for participation? What are the implications of this in terms of informed consent? Does it really matter if potential participants conceive of this money as a direct benefit? Do you think that this could compromise the research?

This case study touches on the differences between 'rules' and 'practice'. You may want to take steps to avoid participants getting into any trouble later for views or experiences they describe, such as asking if the group is willing to maintain confidentiality after the session.

WE DON'T PAY:
'BUS FARES' AND OTHER GIFTS IN RESEARCH

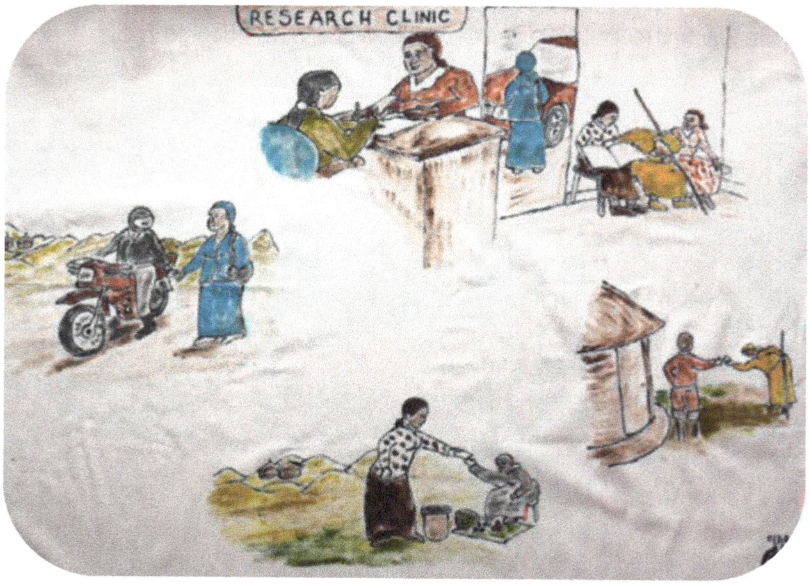

THE PARTICIPANTS HAD DIFFERENT IDEAS ABOUT WHAT TO DO WITH THEIR BUS FARE MONEY

THE STORY

Margaretha is a middle-aged market trader who is participating in a diabetes trial, which aims to improve the management of her condition. She usually walks to the research clinic to attend her scheduled visits. One day, however, one of her legs is more painful than usual, so she contacts the research team and asks for the study vehicle to take her from the market to the research clinic. The research vehicle is not going in that direction, so a fieldworker accompanies her to the clinic by taxi.

After examining her and dressing a wound on her leg, the clinician gives Margaretha a follow-up appointment for the next day, and arranges for her to be collected from the market. Margaretha then goes to the clinic secretary and asks for her usual 'reimbursement' (approximately US$4). The secretary, who has just paid for the taxi, tells her that because she was brought to the clinic by taxi she will not receive this reimbursement today. Margaretha is taken aback, and responds that in that case she does not want a taxi or project vehicle to collect her on the following day. Looking down at the dressing on her painful leg, Margaretha sighs and says, 'Well, I will just have to walk.'

After Margaretha has left the clinic, the secretary goes to see the study coordinator. Feeling bad about refusing the payment, she asks him what she should do. The study coordinator is equally bewildered. The rules concerning transport reimbursement are clear, and although everybody knows that most participants walk to the clinic, it also seems wrong to reimburse somebody whose transport has been paid for by the study. 'But,' says the secretary, 'isn't it wrong to make somebody with a poorly leg walk, especially when that person is your patient?'

A young clinician passes by and throws in an ironic off-hand remark that: 'She waited long enough here before being seen, so isn't she entitled to be paid?'

Upon hearing this, the study coordinator points out that, according to good clinical practice, payments are a form of coercion. 'We can only reimburse participants for travel expenses, nothing else.'

The coordinator telephones the expatriate study PI and she advises that since this is a one off, we should just be kind and pay. The secretary, thinking of her bookkeeping asks the coordinator: 'So what shall I call that payment?'

'Transport reimbursement,' responds her boss, smiling.

QUESTIONS

- What is Margaretha's understanding of 'transport reimbursement'?
- What is the ethical basis of the secretary's argument?
- What do you make of all the other people's views? What ethical beliefs do they express?
- How is the disagreement resolved, and what role do professional hierarchies play in this?

REFLECTION ON YOUR OWN EXPERIENCES

- Can you think of situations in a professional research context, where terms like 'transport reimbursement' is used even though it 'isn't really like that'?
- Can you find other examples, from your experience, where solutions had to be found in practice, rather than through rules?
- Can you think of other situations where senior people resolve dilemmas faced by junior staff through executive decisions, rather than 'by the book'? Who can and should take such decisions? What does this mean for more junior staff?

- What is your experience with modifying or infringing such rules, on a personal level and in relation to your professional responsibilities?

- Can you think of similar situations from your experience – situations in which different positions and experiences, and different understandings of ethics and morality, appeared equally legitimate but hard to reconcile? How did you deal with them? Looking back now, what could you have done differently?

ACTIVITY

Split up into two groups, one group making an argument for reimbursing the participant and the other against. After presenting your opposing arguments to each other, try to find an appropriate solution that will work in practice.

FURTHER READING

Grant, R.W. and Sugarman, J. (2004) Ethics in human subjects research: do incentives matter? *Journal of Medicine and Philosophy* 29(6), 717–738.

Molyneux, S., Mulupi, S., Mbaabu, L., and Marsh, V. (2012) Benefits and payments for research participants: experiences and views from a research centre on the Kenyan coast. *BMC Medical Ethics* 2012 Jun 22, 13:13

YOUR FRIEND HAS NICE CLOTHES:
CONFIDENTIALITY AND STAFF IDENTITY IN HIV HOME FOLLOW-UP

FACILITATOR'S NOTES

This case study is about challenges around confidentiality which can occur when following up with research participants. It talks about how fieldworkers introduce themselves, how they deal with underlying common assumptions and rumours about research, and how they develop relationships and express solidarity with study participants.

When considering the fieldworker's decision to hide her true identity, and the consequences of this or of telling the truth, participants in your group should consider how one's identity as a research worker is associated with many different things: income, project resources, medical expertise, HIV, blood taking (and associated rumours), etc. Some of these could affect people's responses to the fieldworker; others might have effects for the research participant and her relations.

It also raises questions about how research resources are used, by comparing the amount spent on tracing a participant with how this money could have helped this participant meet her child's basic needs. This question might seem pointless, since researchers cannot ignore their responsibility to follow up trial participants. But at the same time it is important to consider how money is spent in research, where savings could be made, and whether these could be directed into support funds for participants in need. This may help address some of the problems fieldworkers face in encountering participants in evident need.

LEARNING OBJECTIVE

To raise awareness of potential challenges – especially regarding confidentiality – when conducting home visits with HIV positive participants, and to discuss the role and personal involvement of research staff in relation to participants

KEYWORDS

Staff identity

Confidentiality

Rumour

Stigma

Home visits

The main focus of this case study, however, is the relationship between fieldworkers and participants – specifically the different identities a fieldworker may adopt in order to establish contact, protect participants' confidentiality, and ensure that they complete the study. It offers the opportunity to discuss these challenges with research staff, allowing them to voice similar problems they may face in their work. This could then lead to thinking about ways research staff can be better supported in carrying out their role.

YOUR FRIEND HAS NICE CLOTHES:
CONFIDENTIALITY AND STAFF IDENTITY IN HIV HOME FOLLOW-UP

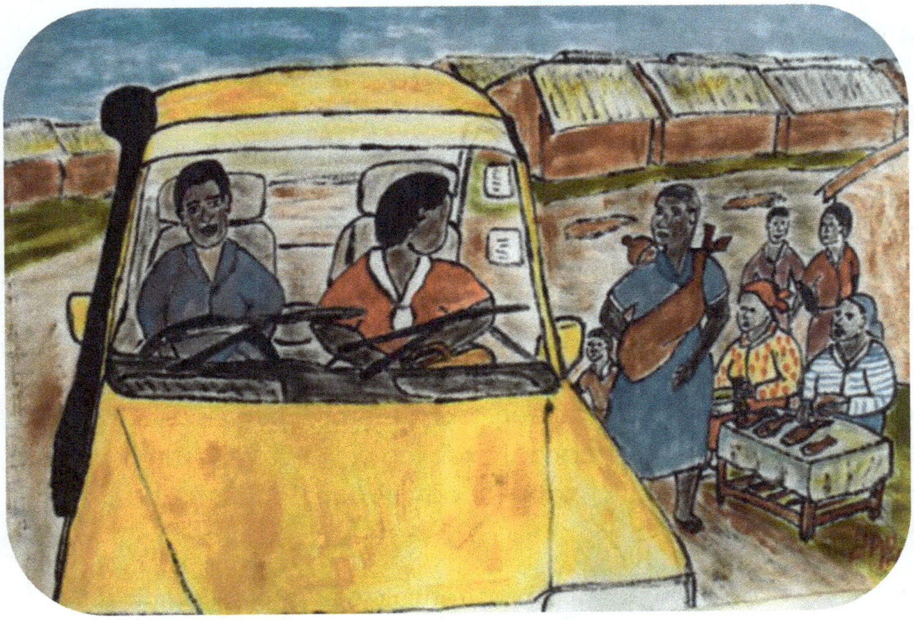

EVERYONE WAS WONDERING WHO WAS CARO'S SMARTLY DRESSED 'FRIEND' WITH THE BIG CAR...

THE STORY

Caro is a young woman and mother, made homeless after her husband rejected her and their baby when he found out that she was HIV positive. Caro has nowhere to go and keeps moving, like many of her fellow research participants on a vaginal microbicide trial. She cannot afford to rent a place of her own; her parents do not want her to return home; and she is also not welcome in her younger sister's marital home. For the time being, she rents a one-room semi-permanent house in a slum area and tries to set up a business selling snacks. Caro has not visited the research clinic for a while and her study visit is overdue.

This is when Maureen gets on the case; her task is to follow-up on lost participants. Caro has no telephone so Maureen has spent two days tracking her through neighbours at her previous address. When asking about Caro's whereabouts in a poor area, several young men start pestering Maureen, on account of her beautiful hair style and clothing. One of the neighbours asks her directly whether the girl she was looking for, Caro, had AIDS.

Happy that she has come with the project Land Rover and the male driver, Maureen sets off towards the opposite side of town, where one of the neighbours claims that Caro lives now. After a lot of discussion, one of the neighbouring women agrees to travel with her and show her the place. When approaching this large and infamous slum, this lady tells Maureen they had better walk, as there is no road to the place. Reluctantly, the driver lets them go, but as they walk he tries to negotiate a way to stay nearby.

The path is muddy and dirty, people look at her dress, and Maureen worries about her handbag. Her guide offers her a plastic bag to hide it from view. Finally they find the place, a small courtyard surrounded by single rooms, in front of each several people and children. Maureen introduces herself and her puzzled guide as Caro's friends from Church fellowship, coming to pray together. Someone goes to fetch Caro from the shops, where she sells chips, but he returns without her, claiming that he did not find her. When Maureen wants to leave again, she finds the Land Rover in front of the compound. Driving off, she spots Caro on the street. They communicate silently with facial gestures and Maureen realises that Caro is afraid of all the questions her neighbours will have about Maureen's presence here.

In low voices, they talk through the car window. Maureen asks general questions about Caro's health, but as Caro refuses to come with her, she cannot examine or weigh her, check her coital diary, or restock her microbicides to check treatment adherence. The forms she brought remain incomplete.

The research team has spent about US$35 on petrol (apart from salaries and allowances for Maureen and the driver) – about the same as Caro's profit from her chips business. In order to encourage Caro to come to the clinic, Maureen gives her money for the bus the next day. From her own pocket she adds some small banknote 'for the children'. Caro hides both in her bra, conscious of the onlookers around her.

QUESTIONS

- Why is Maureen not introducing herself as a research worker on a microbicide study? Should she have done so?
- If she told the truth, what might the implications be for herself, for the research participant, and for the research itself, in the short and long term?
- What do you think the local people, the lady who helps Maureen, and Caro's relatives think about who she is?
- What are the advantages and disadvantages of full openness about one's identity in the field?
- What problems might arise from not revealing one's true identity and purpose?

- What do you think about the use of money in the case study – the resources spent to track Caro, and the personal money that Maureen gives Caro? Is the former an appropriate use of resources, and what does the latter represent?

REFLECTION ON YOUR OWN EXPERIENCES

- In your own research setting, what are the guidelines for fieldworkers when moving around in the field or conducting home visits? Do you think these could be improved upon, and if so, how?

- For your organization, how do local people unrelated to the research project respond to staff?

FURTHER READING

Kamuya, D., Marsh, V., and Molyneux, S. (2011) What we learned about voluntariness and consent: incorporating 'background situations' and understanding into analyses. *The American Journal of Bioethics* 11(8), 31-33. PubMed PMID: 21806436.

Madiega, P.A., Jones, G. et al. (2013). 'She's my sister-In-law, my visitor, my friend' – challenges of staff identity in home follow-up in an HIV trial in Western Kenya. *Developing World Bioethics* 13(1), 21–29.

Simon, C. and Mosavel, M. (2010) Community members as recruiters of human subjects: ethical considerations. *American Journal of Bioethics* 10(3), 3–11.

TRUTH AND LIES:

DOING FIELDWORK IN YOUR OWN COMMUNITY

FACILITATOR'S NOTES

This case study urges us to think carefully about the nuances involved in working as a community-based fieldworker for a research organization. Local assistants are generally highly valued by research organizations because of their insider knowledge, cultural understanding and ability to help researchers gain access and build trust with community members. However, their position as community intermediaries requires them to negotiate complicated issues related to confidentiality and community expectations. In the story below a local fieldworker gains some information which could jeopardize a trial participant's ongoing access to free care. Given her privileged understanding of the situation as a friend and neighbour, she is reluctant to expose the family in question.

This is just one example of some of the dilemmas community-based field assistants can experience as a result of their dual allegiance to their home communities and their employers. Another is spoken and unspoken expectations for material assistance (given their association with a 'wealthy' organization). An additional issue, although it is not really specifically touched on in the story, is that some community members may not feel able to share sensitive information with a fieldworker whom they know very well. For example, they may not want to tell someone who goes to the same church as them that their underage daughter is pregnant. It is important that these nuances are thought through carefully both to support fieldworkers and to ensure that research data is valid and research participants are protected.

In this case, it would be good to get training participants to think about whether and how the trial participant's life could

LEARNING OBJECTIVE

To consider the challenges and dilemmas community-based field assistants can experience as a result of their dual allegiance to their home communities and their employers, and discuss how these could be better addressed

KEYWORDS

Poverty

Study rules

Community-based fieldworkers

Friendship

have been saved. For example, if better follow-up referral processes were in place, would the child's mother, the grandmother, and the fieldworker have been happier to inform the research study about the change in circumstances? In the absence of universal high standards of care, healthcare insurance, or other forms of financial support, there will not be any easy solutions to some of these dilemmas. However, we believe that it is important to bring these dilemmas into the open, in order to share experiences, offer support, and start thinking about how they could be addressed.

TRUTH AND LIES:
DOING FIELDWORK IN YOUR OWN COMMUNITY

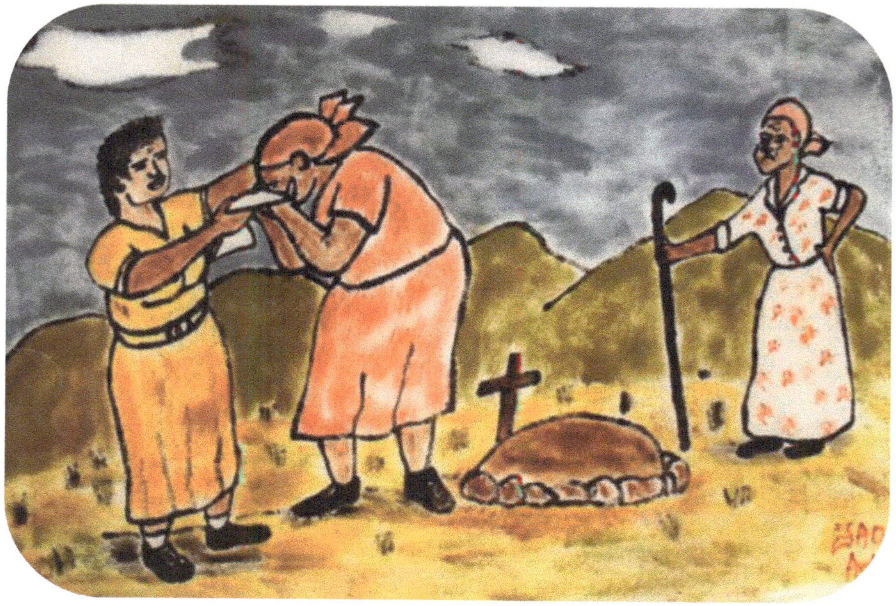

AS SUSAN COMFORTED JUDY'S DAUGHTER SHE WONDERED IF SHE SHOULD HAVE ACTED DIFFERENTLY...

THE STORY

Susan is a community fieldworker for a long-term demographic surveillance project. She works in the village where she has lived since she got married, and is employed on a casual basis to help the demographers keep track of births, deaths and migration. She is regarded as an expert on village relationships by the research organization and is employed for her detailed knowledge of these matters. There is another study ongoing in the area which provides a degree of free healthcare for its participants. It is related to, but not part of, the demographic surveillance project, and Susan does not work on it.

Whilst on one of her regular walk-arounds of the village to check for new births and deaths, Susan meets an old friend, Judy. Judy used to work on the demographic surveillance with Susan a long time ago when the project was being set up. She has a daughter who has a tempestuous relationship with her husband and has been living with her for the last few years. Judy's daughter has a young son who has been sickly from birth and has often benefited from the free treatment provided by the second study.

Judy tells Susan that she is very worried about her daughter, because she has decided to move back to her husband's home under pressure from her in-laws. The home is outside the catchment area of the study and this will mean that Judy's grandson will no longer benefit from the free treatment.

A few weeks later Susan is surprised to see Judy's daughter and grandson at the local study hospital. Judy's grandson is seriously ill and has been admitted, but there is some confusion about who will pay the bill. The researchers suspect that Judy's daughter has left home. They ask Susan for confirmation. Susan knows that Judy and her daughter don't have the resources to pay the bill and she is not 100 per cent sure that Judy's daughter has really left home, given the tempestuous relationship she has with her husband. She tells the researchers she 'thinks' Judy's daughter still resides in the village. Later, Susan talks to Judy about it and Judy tells her that she is just 'keeping quiet' when the researchers ask about changes in who lives in her home. After all, who knows how long her daughter will stay with her husband this time?

Susan does not work on the free treatment study and is unsure what to do. Judy is a good friend and she is concerned she will lose her trust if she tells the researchers her daughter has moved out. Susan is also concerned about Judy's grandson's welfare. She knows Judy's daughter's husband and considers him a 'bad' man who will not look after them well. She decides to think about the issue for a while.

A few weeks later Susan hears from Judy that her grandson is sick again, but that her son-in-law is refusing to take him to the nearest hospital because he can get free treatment in the study hospital. But Judy's daughter doesn't have money to pay the fare to take him to her mother's village. Judy asks Susan to lend her the money, which she does. But by this time, her grandson is dangerously dehydrated. He is admitted to the study hospital for over a week but sadly does not recover.

Susan attends the funeral, which is held at Judy's home. Judy's daughter and her husband have separated for good this time.

QUESTIONS

- What are the challenges identified here, for both Susan and the study?
- What do you think Susan could have done differently? Do you think the outcome would have been the same?
- In these kinds of circumstances, what are the advantages and disadvantages of working in the place you live, from the worker's and employer's perspective? How about from the perspective of local people in the community – in what ways does it help, and in what ways does it get in the way to have your friends employed as fieldworkers?

- Do you think that Judy's grandson should have remained eligible for study benefits even though he had moved out of catchment? Please explain your reasons either way.
- Why do you think Judy asks Sarah to lend her some money? Could this have anything to do with her work, or is it just a neighbourly request?
- What bigger issues shape this story? What are the background challenges which contribute to the death of the little boy?

REFLECTION ON YOUR OWN EXPERIENCE:

Have you experienced or witnessed similar scenarios in the course of your work? If yes, how did you, or others, manage these kinds of issues?

FURTHER READING

Chantler, T., Otewa, F. et al. (2013) Ethical challenges that arise at the community interface of health research: village reporters' experiences in Western Kenya. *Developing World Bioethics* 13(1), 30–37.

Kamuya, D.M., Theobald, S.J. et al. (2013) Evolving friendships and shifting ethical dilemmas: fieldworkers' experiences in a short term community based study in Kenya. *Developing World Bioethics* 13(1), 1–9.

Simon, C. and Mosavel, M. (2010) Community members as recruiters of human subjects: ethical considerations. *American Journal of Bioethics* 10(3), 3–11.

I COULD BE A SEX WORKER:

MEANINGS OF EXCLUSION AND INCLUSION CRITERIA TO PARTICIPANTS

FACILITATOR'S NOTES

Sometimes researchers complain about participants being dishonest or lying in order to 'greedily' get into trials, and participants' motives are labelled as 'good' or 'bad'. However, the poor quality of public healthcare available in some places and the wider context of global health inequality make it difficult to pass judgment on participants' attempts to obtain treatment. Inclusion criteria for trials matter to researchers from the point of view of funding and scientific rigour, but for participants, they can be a matter of life or death.

This case study asks training groups to put themselves in the shoes of a participant who is keen to get onto a project. Whatever their final verdict on her actions, hopefully discussing the case will help them to understand her. You may want to emphasize how confusing the various options for care might seem to participants, and how they often need to become adept at representing themselves and their condition in order to navigate this complex landscape. The story is about accessing post-trial care, but from a patient's point of view, this is not particularly important. The same issues could arise around recruitment to a research project.

The story also points towards several wider issues which your group may like to reflect upon: what is 'fair' in the context of global health inequality; specific cultural attitudes towards what counts as 'sex work'; and the potential dynamics between researchers and study participants.

LEARNING OBJECTIVE

To reflect on differences between how research participants and study coordinators may view inclusion criteria, and to appreciate the reasons behind this

KEYWORDS

Recruitment

Post-trial care

Inclusion and exclusion criteria

Standards of Care

Money

I COULD BE A SEX WORKER:
MEANINGS OF EXCLUSION AND INCLUSION CRITERIA TO PARTICIPANTS

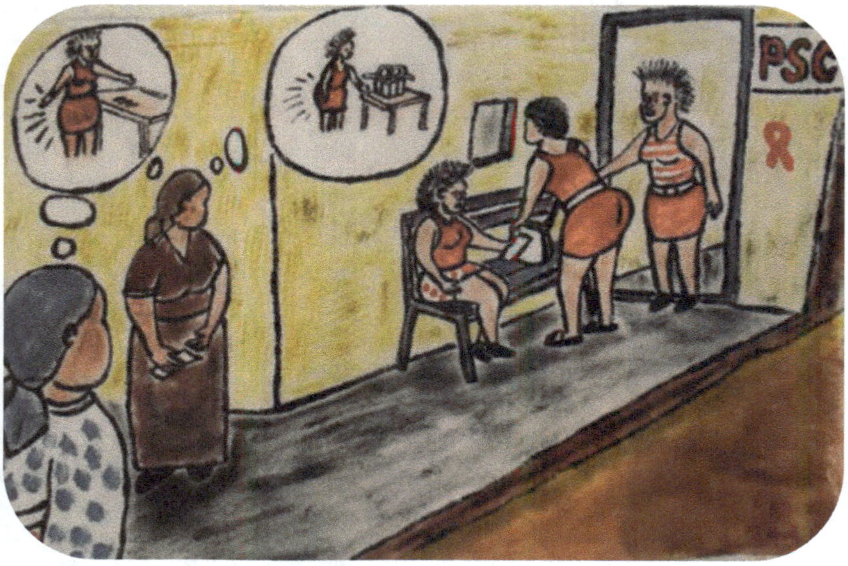

MAUREEN THOUGHT, 'OK, IF I GET MYSELF SOME TIGHTER CLOTHES I COULD BE A SEX WORKER...'

THE STORY

In this busy African city there are several large transnational medical research organizations, and many NGOs providing a range of care and treatment services for people living with HIV/AIDS.

Maureen is an HIV positive woman who has just exited a research study looking at the progression of HIV and Hepatitis B co-infections. During her time in the study she received her HIV care and treatment at a study clinic. She felt she received excellent care, as well as having her transport to the clinic reimbursed. She also enjoyed being a member of an active self-help group, and attending several training sessions for which she received certificates. Before exiting the study Maureen and the other participants are advised to think carefully about where they would like to receive their care and treatment post-research.

Maureen has done her research well on the options available to her. She has visited the various clinics and spoken to other research participants who have already exited the study. She decides that the best place for her is a clinic run by a Swedish organization which caters specifically for commercial sex workers. One of the friends she made during her time in the study, a sex worker in a local bar, has told her that if she 'gets a spot' in the clinic she'll continue to get her transport reimbursed, and that there may be employment opportunities there for her as a peer educator. The only problem is that Maureen has not considered herself to be a sex worker before now. She has had a number of boyfriends and concurrent relationships, but actual money has not changed hands. Her sex worker friend tells her this shouldn't matter. She advises her to say that she is a sex worker with a number of 'long-term clients' or 'sugar daddies', rather than short-term engagements. She also tells her to say that one of her boyfriends (or 'clients') pays the monthly rent on her house. This, she advises, will help her qualify.

Maureen goes for an interview at the sex workers' clinic. She wears a little more make-up than usual and copies the dressing style of her friend. Her friend gives her a 'peer referral' to the clinic as well. Maureen is accepted at the clinic and also joins the self-help group. A few months later, Maureen applies for, and gets, one of the highly sought-after peer educator positions. Her certificates and training from the former study, as well as her ambition and commitment, have impressed the interviewers.

QUESTIONS

- What do you think about what Maureen does? Why does she do it? What do you think the consequences might be for Maureen, and for the organization?
- Why do you think the Swedish organization is only open to 'sex workers'? Do you think this is important from the point of view of people living with HIV/AIDS?
- Do you think it is important to Maureen that the first organization she receives care from is a research project and the second an NGO?
- Do you think Maureen will make a good HIV peer educator?
- Can you think of anything that could help avoid this type of situation?
- If you were a member of staff in the Swedish organization and you found out that Maureen does not think of herself as a sex worker, what would you do?
- Is it always clear what 'sex work' is?
- Is this situation also applicable to participation in research studies?
- What do you think this story tells us about how the presence of overseas organizations may be interacting with local culture?

- What could you say about the wider issues behind this situation? Do you think the overseas organizations are doing a good job?
- 'Sex work' suggests making a living from your body. Do you think this story can tell us anything about the interaction between medical organizations and research participants?

REFLECTIONS ON YOUR OWN EXPERIENCE

- Have you ever been in a situation like this where boundaries have been blurred (either as a member of staff, or changing the way you represent yourself to get something you need)? How did you approach the situation? What happened?
- Have you experienced similar situations in recruiting research participants for studies?

FURTHER READING

Aellah, G. and Geissler, P.W (2016) Seeking exposure: conversions of scientific knowledge in an African City: *The Journal of Modern African Studies* 54(3) pp 389-417

Geissler, P.W. (2013) Stuck in ruins, or up and coming? The shifting geography of urban public health research in Kisumu, Kenya. *Africa: Journal of the International African Institute* 83, 539–560.

Prince, R. (2012) HIV and the moral economy of survival in an East African city. *Medical Anthropology Quarterly* 26(4), 534–556.

Simon, C. and Mosavel, M. (2010) Community members as recruiters of human subjects: ethical considerations. *American Journal of Bioethics* 10(3) 3–11.

THEY JUST COME AND ASK QUESTIONS:
PARTICIPANTS' UNDERSTANDINGS OF THE PURPOSE OF RESEARCH

FACILITATOR'S NOTES

This case study invites us to consider challenges which can arise from the involvement of households in long-term demographic surveillance systems. Such systems represent an invaluable resource for researchers conducting studies which aim to assess the effectiveness of new healthcare interventions. In the long term, this research may also have direct benefits for household members who provide demographic information. However, the value of this research can seem less evident to them in the short term, and, as we read in this story, some of the questions which are asked as part of surveillance activities can give rise to misplaced hopes or expectations for material help.

The aim of the story is to serve as a catalyst for discussions about consent processes in this type of research, and ways of addressing misunderstandings about the purpose of demographic surveillance. In terms of consent, it is important to think about the way households are organized with reference to cultural norms. In the rural community portrayed here it is usual for newly married women to live with their husbands in a larger compound, which can include several houses. The owner of the compound is the father-in-law, and so he is the decision-maker when it comes to who is welcome in the compound. He must consent for the fieldworkers to visit his compound before any of the other compound members are approached. However, given the long-term nature of the demographic surveillance activities a case could be made for renewing this consent on an annual basis.

LEARNING OBJECTIVE

To consider challenges that can arise in the conduct of long-term research projects which involve health and demographic surveillance and do not result in short-term benefits

KEYWORDS

Informed consent

Long-term engagement

Comprehension

Poverty

In addition, there is a need to ensure that all household members are given information about the purpose of collecting demographic data and any possible benefits. Encourage your training participants to think about ways this could be achieved, and how they would explain the purpose of the demographic surveillance system and the reasons for including questions about household assets. You could also ask participants to consider why community members may find it difficult to distinguish between research and development organizations, and how this misconception could be addressed. If you are based at a research centre which is involved in demographic surveillance, try to find out more about how this works before the session. It would also be a good idea to review the types of questions asked during fieldwork, and to think about how these might be viewed by community members.

THEY JUST COME AND ASK QUESTIONS:

PARTICIPANTS' UNDERSTANDINGS OF THE PURPOSE OF RESEARCH

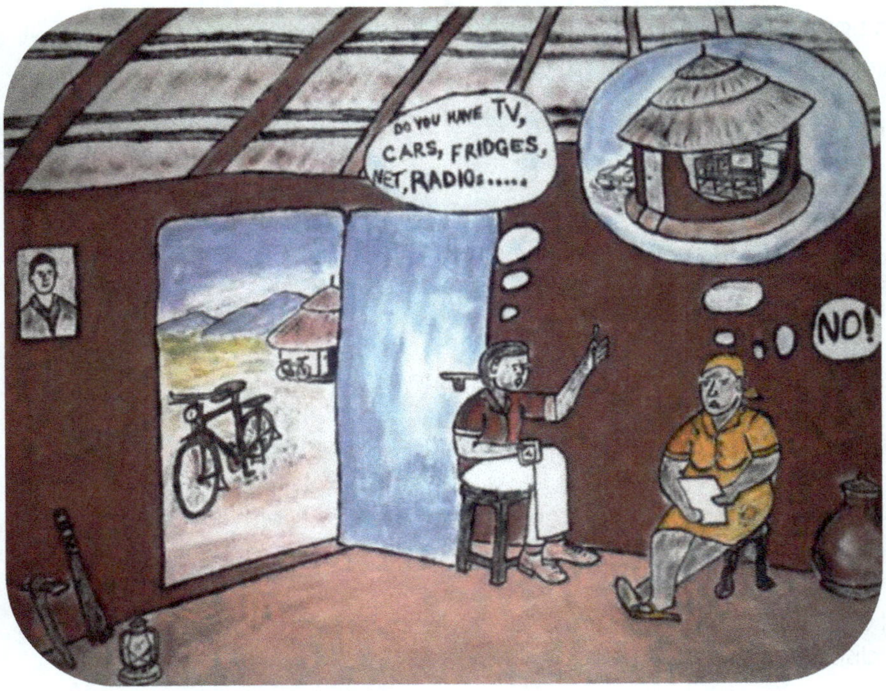

'MY HUT IS GOING TO BE AMAZING!' THOUGHT JESSIE. 'I WONDER WHEN HE'LL BRING ALL THESE NEW THINGS?'

THE STORY

A demographic surveillance system has been functioning in a rural area for many years. Every three months, fieldworkers visit homes and compounds in the area and ask household members about who has moved in and out, and whether there have been any births or deaths. Sometimes they ask about possessions owned by household members including bicycles, cows, televisions and thermos flasks. The homes were originally included into the system after consent had been obtained from the head of each household, who provided permission on behalf of all the other household members. Many years on the community has become very used to both the fieldworkers and the questions.

Jessie recently moved into the area after marrying the son of one of the household heads. The next time the fieldworker visits, Jessie is the only person at home. The fieldworker, Jim, arrives by bicycle. This is the 15th household he has visited today and he has many more to visit. Jim introduces himself briefly and starts asking Jessie his questions on behalf of the whole household. Jessie's husband told her something like this would happen so she is not surprised. When Jim starts asking her about number of bicycles they have, she answers none, although this isn't true. She does not show it, but in her heart she is quite excited. She thinks that perhaps this is a non-governmental organization doing a survey of things that are needed in their household, and hopes they might bring them next time. She has heard that there are lots of NGOs operating in this area.

When Jessie's husband gets home she tells him all about it. He tells her, no, they never bring those things. 'Oh,' says Jessie, 'then why are they asking the questions?'

'Hmm,' says her husband. 'I'm not sure.'

QUESTIONS

- Why do you think the head of the household was the one who was asked to provide consent on behalf of all the residents?
- Why do you think Jessie kept quiet, even if she was excited?
- Why do you think Jim did not explain the purpose of the research to her?
- Why do you think Jessie thought the fieldworker might come back with some things for the home?
- What does all this tell us about how participants and researchers view each other, even though it is not really discussed?
- Why do you think Jessie's husband could not answer her questions? What does this tell us about the ethical position of the project?
- What do you think the consequences of this misunderstanding could be? Is it a big deal?
- How well could you answer Jessie's question?
- Do you think it is possible or desirable to keep re-consenting? What are some of the drawbacks?
- What strategies could be put in place to help this situation?

REFLECTION ON YOUR OWN EXPERIENCES

- What other situations does this remind you of?
- Is this different from therapeutic misconception? What are the similarities and differences?
- This case study shows that it is important to understand local structures of authority, respect and consenting when doing research, but that this can also be challenging for achieving individual consent and understanding. What other examples of this do you have from your own work?

FURTHER READING

Carrel, M. and Rennie, S. (2008) Demographic and health surveillance: longitudinal ethical considerations. *Bulletin of the World Health Organization* 86(8), 612–616.

Mondain, N. (2010) Exploring respondents' understanding and perceptions of demographic surveillance systems in Western Africa: methodological and ethical issues. *African Population Studies* 24(3), 149–165.

RESPONSIBILITY FOR WHAT AND WHOM?:

END-OF-TRIAL AND LONG-TERM HEALTHCARE

FACILITATOR'S NOTES

This case study is about researchers' responsibilities towards study participants beyond the end of a trial. Three main issues are likely to arise in discussions: researchers' general responsibility for follow-up after the end of trial; their responsibility for follow-up when access to appropriate treatment is poor in the public health system; and the legal and ethical responsibility of both researchers and their sponsors to follow up participants whose health is placed at risk as a result of the trial. Before you use this case study you may want to check up on the legal requirements for research in your setting, and think about how these are applied in the studies conducted at your site.

In the questions at the end of this case study, certain terms are used which you might need to unpack for your students. 'Legal liability' would mean researchers' responsibility for any negative effects of the trial, which can be proven formally to arise directly from patients' participation. Both 'personal' and 'institutional' responsibility can be linked to legal liability (national or international), but can also be thought of as being independent of direct causation. They arise through long-term engagement with the participants, and are also influenced by the availability of resources that could help in a specific situation.

'Feasibility', 'justice' and 'equity', on the other hand, are 'macro' concepts which require students to consider the wider context of the research. Exploring these ideals might lead students to suggest that, given how much it would cost to

LEARNING OBJECTIVE

To explore researchers' responsibility towards study participants beyond the course of a trial, and to discuss differences between organizational responsibility, personal obligation and legal liability

KEYWORDS

Post-trial care

Clinical responsibility

Standards of care

Long-term engagement

Research versus care

follow-up all participants in the trial, these resources would be better used for wider public health aims, benefiting a larger population. This case study then points to a discussion about the role of rich international research organizations within poor countries, and the relationship between scientific and political engagement.

RESPONSIBILITY FOR WHAT AND WHOM?:

END-OF-TRIAL AND LONG-TERM HEALTHCARE

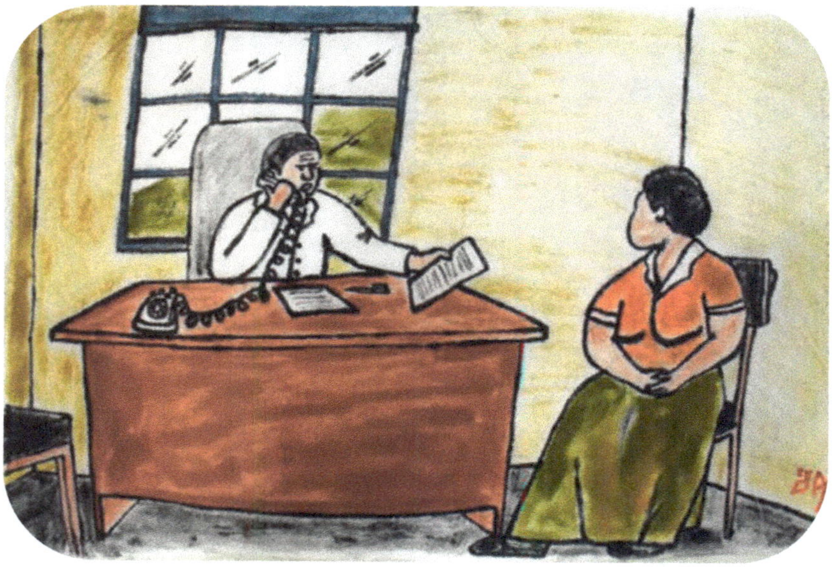

.'SO….YOUR RESEARCH PROJECT WANTS ME TO DO WHAT?!'

THE STORY

A trial of a new drug regime for the treatment of Hepatitis B enrols men and women with chronic infections. The drugs are tested and approved internationally, but are not usually given as routine treatment in this African country due to their cost and the unreliability of supplies. In the study, the drugs are given for one year. Participants are then 'exited' from the research and referred to local hospitals for continued monitoring.

When they are referred on, participants are given a letter containing information on their health status and recommendations on how their infections should be monitored. The letters all state that it would be good for the participants to be kept on the trial drug regime for longer, if local resources allow. Aware that this may be difficult, the researchers make recommendations about carefully considered alternative treatments, and provide a contact number for the new doctors to call to discuss this further. Researchers advise the participants to try to find treatment at a larger hospital in the nearby city, which has specialist Hepatitis B care and good links with the research organization.

However, many of the participants prefer to seek treatment in the small clinics near their home villages, due to transport costs and their familiarity with the staff. Now that they are no longer receiving transport allowances through the study, many participants cannot afford a long trip. When the participants take their letters to the smaller clinics, some of the resident clinical officers there are unable to interpret the information. Some of the clinicians admit this, but others tell the ex-participants that they are unhappy at 'being told what to do' by foreign scientists 'who don't know this place'. Sometimes the clinicians at the small centres contact the trial clinicians and are given further advice. One of them even uses the opportunity to visit the research centre to update his knowledge.

Hepatitis B care is still under development in this region and not all clinics have access to the latest drugs and tests. Although, officially, relevant drugs should be available in local clinics, this is not usually the case. A widely publicized report by an international NGO draws attention to this problem. Some of the ex-participants' cases are then resolved through personal interventions by the research clinicians, who know whom to call at the national drug procurement programme to get them to send adequate supplies to a particular centre.

The researchers soon realize that it would be good to continue to monitor what happens to the trial participants over the coming years, and they apply for funding from their organization to help them maintain contact. They start to find that a few of the participants have developed resistance to the drugs, and theorize this is because of the interruption in their treatment when they leave the study.

However, finding all the participants after the end of the trial and communicating with them is not always easy or cheap. Most of them have had only primary school education, sometimes unfinished; some of them are single mothers; hardly any has regular work or employment; few have a permanent residence. As a result of economic and social insecurity, many move between different urban locations, their parents' and other relatives' rural homes, or their marital homes. Such moves either require regular transport back to their local clinic, which few can afford, or transfer the patients from one clinic to another, requiring lots of paperwork, the involvement of new doctors, and time lost in trial periods.

The case of these participants creates debates among doctors, scientists and managers involved in the trial. Some feel that the study should have continued to provide drugs directly to the smaller centres for those participants whom they felt would benefit. Others argue that the participants' Hepatitis B infections will not be properly monitored in the smaller clinics. Many of the researchers feel concerned about the fate of the participants they have become close to over the course of the trial.

QUESTIONS

- If you were a researcher on this study, how do you think you would feel? Do you think your feelings should be reflected in the policy of the organization?

- What role do each of the issues below play in this case? Who is responsible for implementing each of them?

    1. Legal-medical liability (under local or international law)
    2. Personal and institutional responsibility and morality
    3. Concerns with feasibility and equity

- What would post-trial plans look like if the researchers prioritized:

    1. Obligations/responsibilities on the individual level?
    2. Justice/feasibility, for everybody or at the population level?
    3. Liability, legal obligation, or economic risk at the managerial level?

- What different perspectives do you think different people might have on this issue? You might want to consider the possible views of participants, workers in the local healthcare facilities, people working at the national drug procurement programme, research fieldworkers/nurses, study coordinators, scientists, funding bodies, and in-country government officials (local and national)?

- Do you think calls for the highest possible standards of care and continued responsibility are justified? What is the impact of such demands on individual research projects?

REFLECTION ON YOUR OWN EXPERIENCES

- What happens to research participants in your work when they leave a study and are referred to public hospitals? What has this meant for you, personally?

- What limitations are implied by your organization about its responsibility for further care?

- What do you think your organization could do to support local healthcare? For example, does it provide clear and up-to-date information on drugs and future treatment options available? Does it engage with the practicalities of this – how much it might cost, and how it might support local clinics to follow the recommendations?

FURTHER READING

de Cenival, M. (2008) L'éthique de la recherche ou la liberté d'en sortir [Ethics of research : the freedom to withdraw]. *Bulletin of the Exotic Pathology Society* 101(2), 98–101.

Shaffer, D. N. et al. (2006) Equitable treatment for HIV/AIDS clinical trial participants: A focus group study of patients, clinician researchers, and administrators in Western Kenya. *Journal of Medical Ethics* 32.1: 55–60.

HUNGER IS NOT OUR MANDATE:

DEALING WITH POVERTY AMONG RESEARCH PARTICIPANTS

FACILITATOR'S NOTES

This story is about how far people conducting scientific research among poor populations decide whether to allow poverty – and more specifically hunger – to come under the remit of their activities. Here, in a research project involving children and their parents from a poor area, participants and staff do not talk about the fact that many of the children are hungry, and many of the parents worry about not finding food for them. The absence of discussion about the subject is striking because the subject of the research is nutrition and weight.

The story sheds light on a question that appears in many similar situations: how can one, as a research worker, relate to the poverty of the people one meets through research? While the researchers here are clearly concerned about nutrition – it is the rationale for their research – it is harder to consider how this affects them personally. The question is what responsibilities arise from the encounter between relatively privileged researchers, and research participants with essential needs?

Various questions may emerge. Does economic inequality have anything to do with the research? Or is it a private matter, separate from science? If so, how do researchers reconcile private experiences and responsibilities with their professional roles? How does this sit with ethics rules about non-inducement, and scientific standards of objective research? Or should research take on a wider responsibility when engaging people who lack essentials such as food or medicine? If so, how, and funded by whom? What are the limits to this responsibility? Who decides, and how?

LEARNING OBJECTIVE

To reflect upon poverty among research participants and how far medical research can and should address this

KEYWORDS

Research versus care

Long- term engagement

Poverty

Post-trial care

HUNGER IS NOT OUR MANDATE:
DEALING WITH POVERTY AMONG RESEARCH PARTICIPANTS

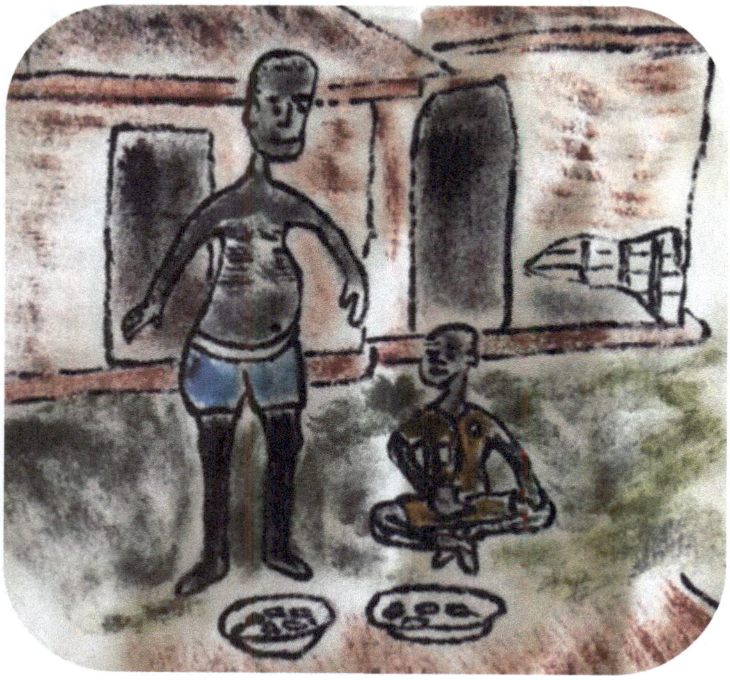

'NO. TODAY WE DID NOT EAT ICE-CREAM.'

THE STORY

For a study on gastrointestinal infections and weight gain, primary school children from an urban slum are recruited and asked to visit a clinic regularly with their caregivers. They are also invited to visit the clinic in the case of any illness and provided with free treatment. Apart from this, staff are cautioned by supervisors not to provide any 'material incentives' to research participants, because such gestures could potentially infringe ethical regulations.

Part of the regular appointments is a 'food frequency' questionnaire, filled out after weighing the children and taking measurements. The questionnaire asks how regularly and in which quantities the children eat particular foods. The five-page list of foods is taken from a standard nutritional assessment tool, and ranges from maize to ice-cream, from cabbage to yoghurt. The survey is completed by a '24-hour recall diet' recording, which asks children about the food and drink they have consumed in the past day. It assumes children have had three regular meals and up to four intermediate snacks. Although the children are supposed to answer the questions, the accompanying caregivers usually help with the task.

When answering the questionnaire, the children occasionally ask questions about foods mentioned in the questionnaire which they don't know. Otherwise, they do their best to answer all the questions put to them by the nutritional counsellor truthfully. They do not mention the obvious difference between the range of foods mentioned in the questions (which are sometimes expensive), or the way the questionnaire assumes they have regular meals (plus snacks!), and their own everyday realities. Their answers usually include very few basic foods, and frequently skipped meals.

However, while the participants are waiting outside for their appointments, unattended by staff, they speak with each other about this. Sometimes they joke about the questions the counsellors ask, which are so far from their lived realities: 'How can she ask me whether I eat ice cream and bread?!'

This gap is not addressed by the research staff either, although from the regular home visits and from simply living in the same city they are familiar with slum residents' economic situation. Sometimes, when talking privately and among trusted colleagues, they express sympathy with participants' misery, and they commonly give small amounts of their own money or bring food or old clothes on home visits for participants who are obviously needy.

One word in particular that does not appear anywhere in the questionnaire is 'hunger'. Only very rarely, one of the children's parents mentions that finding the means to feed children is a challenge, and asks for support. Usually this happens not in the clinic but during home visits, when staff and participants establish more personal relationships. (The children's parents are, of course, aware that the staff earn good salaries.) Staff never discuss participants' requests, nor their own responses, in formal meetings, or when talking to their supervisors.

When asked why hunger is nowhere on the questionnaire, the clinic staff are quick to point out that 'this would be embarrassing for the women'. The Principal Investigator of a breastfeeding study which is taking place in the same area, however, answers more fully: 'Hunger is a background reality for everybody here; poverty forms the backdrop of all our research here. But it is outside the remit of the research project. Hunger is a matter of development aid programmes, and not of scientific institutions; it is not our mandate. I cannot fund measures against hunger through my research budget.'

QUESTIONS

- Why is the participants' hunger not directly spoken about in the meetings at the clinic between staff and participants? Why can it be discussed when research staff visit participants, or when either participants or research staff are 'among themselves'?
- Why did the supervisor advise research staff not to give participants food or money? Discuss the various possible consequences of doing this. Do you think it worth the risk?
- If hunger were mentioned more explicitly, who would be embarrassed and why?
- The overseas Principal Investigator gives different reasons from the clinic staff about why hunger is not mentioned. What do you think of her explanation? Do you think she cares about people on the project? From what she says, what can we understand about her beliefs and culture?
- What do you think about the fact that it is local staff who end up paying money and giving clothes to the participants, not the project itself or the overseas staff? In what ways is this fair or right, and in what ways not?
- What do you think are the potential advantages and disadvantages of talking more about hunger and poverty?
- What else could this research organization do to support its staff?

REFLECTION ON YOUR OWN EXPERIENCES

- How is poverty, especially that of research participants, discussed in your research setting?
- When are words like 'poverty' or 'hunger' – terms that describe gross inequalities or actual economic misery – used in your research setting? How do they feature in publications and minutes of research meetings? What does this tell us?
- When, and with whom, can one talk about these issues in your organization, and with whom would one avoid these subjects? Why?
- Are there subjects which people (at any level) joke about in your organization, but which aren't mentioned in other places? Do you think anything could or should be done about these issues?

FURTHER READING

Kalofonos, I.A. (2010) 'All I eat is ARVs': the paradox of AIDS treatment interventions in Central Mozambique. *Medical Anthropology Quarterly* 24(3), 363–380.

Prince, R. (2012) HIV and the moral economy of survival in an East African city. *Medical Anthropology Quarterly* 26(4), 534–556.

THEY JUST WANT TO SIGN QUICKLY:

DIFFERENT INTERPRETATIONS OF INFORMED CONSENT

FACILITATOR'S NOTES

This case study is about different understandings of the informed consent process and the documents associated with it. Here, four different approaches to informed consent within a study open up multiple overlapping interpretations of what it may mean.

You can use this case study as a springboard for discussion, looking at who holds each view – participants, fieldworkers, research designers, external commentators, etc. Each of these 'groups' is not necessarily a single unit; people within them may hold multiple overlapping or conflicting perspectives. In trying to unpick these interpretations, you may need to encourage your group to look at all of them as equally valid, rather than factually 'correct' or 'wrong'. A medical-legal model of consent, or a scientific one, after all, is just another cultural view.

Some of the understandings described here may include viewing the consent process and documents as:

- An entry-point to cash and healthcare benefits
- A way to address social injustice
- A way to avoid unethical and abusive practices
- An agreement between researchers and study participants, involving mutual obligations and entitlements
- An absolute principle which, once included in any form, guarantees sound scientific data
- A starting-point for interpretation about what is 'fair'

LEARNING OBJECTIVE

To understand different interpretations of the informed consent process among researchers, social scientists, and participants, and to reflect on how to deal with withdrawals, silent refusals, and avoidance ethically

KEYWORDS

Inducements

Informed consent

Documents

- A way of recognising the autonomy of individuals to make decisions
- A highly social practice, in which powerful authorities recruit newcomers into the project via a ritual induction ceremony
- A document conveying status and prestige

Before using this case study, think carefully about how it relates to current views and practice in your organization, how it might challenge them, and how to protect those taking part in your discussion. You may want to take steps such as asking if the group wants to declare the meeting a confidential and 'safe' space to discuss this important principle.

THEY JUST WANT TO SIGN QUICKLY:
DIFFERENT INTERPRETATIONS OF INFORMED CONSENT

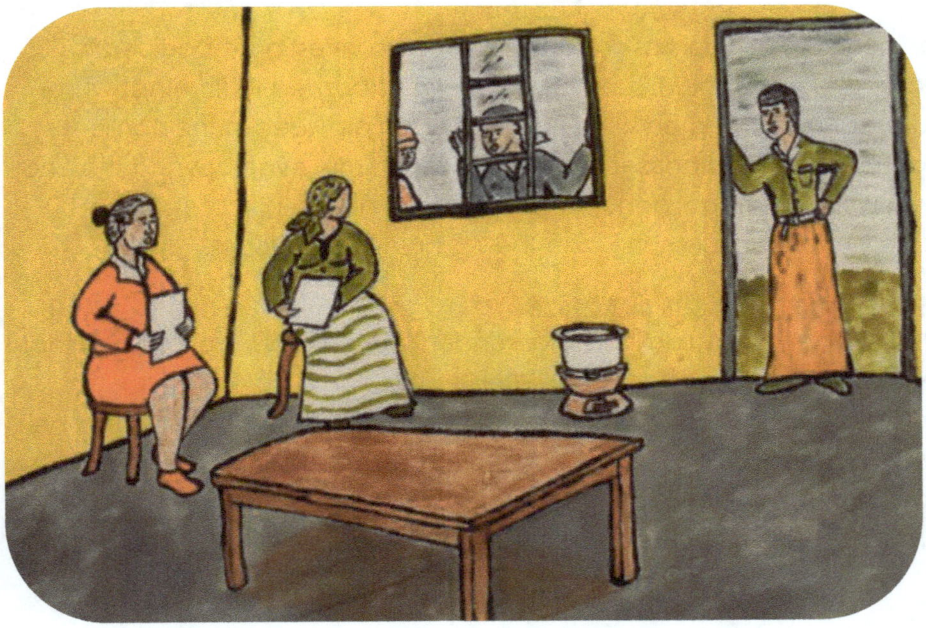

THE PARTICIPANTS FOUND EVERYTHING ELSE MORE INTERESTING THAN THE CONSENT FORMS.

THE STORIES

VOLUNTARY OR INDUCED CONSENT?
Guideline 7 of the Council for International Organizations of Medical Sciences (CIOMS) states that 'Subjects may be reimbursed for lost earnings, travel costs and other expenses incurred in taking part in a study; they may also receive free medical services [...] The payments should not be so large, however, or the medical services so extensive as to induce prospective subjects to consent to participate in the research against their better judgment ("undue inducement").'

A three-year sexual health research project involving 1000 participants is taking place in a city slum in Chad. All participants must sign a consent form on enrolment to the study. The consent form states that: 'Medical care for common medical problems will be given to you and your immediate family at the study clinic at no cost while you are in the study'. Later on in the consent form it states: 'Participation in this study is voluntary. You are not obliged to participate in this study, and even if you agree to participate today, you can change your mind later. If you do so, you will not have disadvantage from this.'

CONSENT AS DOCUMENT OR RITUAL?

Fieldworkers from the city slum project feel that the research participants 'do not take consent seriously at all'. They report that during the study's 'information and consent' sessions, people appear bored when the forms are read out to them; others glance at them but do not seem to pay much attention when doing so. Fieldworkers comment that 'most of them just want to sign the papers quickly and proceed to the clinic'.

Concerned by this trend, the trial managers ask a social scientist to investigate participants' perspectives on informed consent. The social scientist is somewhat puzzled to find that while participants do indeed appear unconcerned with the information provided in the consent process, many of them keep their signed consent forms for a long time, even beyond the end of the trial. They store them with other legal documents, contracts and certificates. One person even framed her consent form and hung it on the wall in her living room.

WITHDRAWING CONSENT – PRINCIPLE VERSUS PRACTICE

The commentary to CIOMS Guideline 7 guideline states, under 'Withdrawal from a study', that 'A subject who withdraws from research for reasons related to the study, such as unacceptable side effects of a study drug, or who is withdrawn on health grounds, should be paid or recompensed as if full participation had taken place. A subject who withdraws for any other reason should be paid in proportion to the amount of participation. An investigator who must remove a subject from the study for willful noncompliance is entitled to withhold part or all of the payment.'

Under a section on 'Withdrawing from the Study,' the consent form for the city slum project states that 'If you withdraw later, you will not suffer any negative consequences'.

As part of this study, as well as routinely taking blood for testing, frequent penile swabs are taken from male participants. Many of the men find the experience uncomfortable and embarrassing. Once these start, numerous participants who have signed consent forms deny field staff access to their homes, or do not show up for their scheduled monthly clinic visits. But a minority of these people continue to seek care and medication from the trial clinic at times of illness. Others still bring their children to the clinic, although they themselves are not complying with study procedures.

The wave of non-compliance and withdrawal threatens the validity of the overall study, and leads to discussions among trial managers, scientists and staff about possible solutions. One nurse reports that, in a different study, he refused to provide care to families of participants who had withdrawn or were no longer complying. Some of his colleagues wonder whether this is right. 'Is it really the children's fault if the father refuses? Shouldn't we continue to provide treatment for the children at least?' The study coordinator interjects: 'I can see your point, but if we provided treatment for everybody, even if they refused the swabs, then who would *choose* to participate in the trial?'

The discussion soon moves on to possible solutions. So few of the participants are actually returning to the trial clinic after their first swab that the study staff decide that free healthcare is no longer going to work as an incentive for people to take part.

CONSENT AS EXCHANGE?

The social scientist involved in the city slum project visits some of non-compliant participants at home, to ask why they have not been attending scheduled visits. She visits the home of a participant who has not brought any family members to the clinic for routine treatment either. When she asks why the family no longer access the clinic's superior healthcare services, the participant's wife replies: 'How can you break an agreement and yet you want to continue to be paid? Can you offend your host and still want to eat his food? If you are part of research, you have to give your blood.'

QUESTIONS

- Why do you think people appear bored when signing the consent form?
- Who do you think is not taking consent seriously?
- What do you think the meaning of signatures on contracts might be in a community where many people can't read? Why do you think study participants keep their consent forms?
- The study design suggests that consent is something freely given by an empowered person. Do you think this is how everyone on the project views it? What other views are there?
- What different understandings are present among research staff and trial participants, and in the guidelines and the consent form, about trial-related healthcare provision?
- Do you think trial-related healthcare is 'undue inducement'?
- What would you do if you were the staff, deciding whether to provide healthcare to non-compliant participants and their families? Why?
- Who do you think should interpret how much people should be 'paid' who withdraw? How might this work if there is no money, just trial-related healthcare?
- What might you do differently if you were working on this project, to minimize the problems of withdrawal?

REFLECTION ON YOUR OWN EXPERIENCES

- What is the practice where you work concerning non-compliant participants or withdrawals: do they receive continued free healthcare? Are there other benefits that they continue or do not continue to access?
- Have the reasons for this ever been discussed on your project? If not, why do you think that such debates do not commonly take place?
- How 'free' do you think participants are in medical research projects which target poor populations? In what ways do you think people express any freedom?

ACTIVITY

Form two groups. One prepares arguments in favour of continued care for non-compliant participants; the other assembles arguments for discontinuation of care. Make sure you include both practical arguments as well as ethical considerations.

FURTHER READING

Council for International Organizations of Medical Sciences (2002) CIOMS Guidelines. Available at: http://www.cioms.ch/publications/guidelines/guidelines_nov_2002_blurb.htm (accessed 25 October 2015).

Leach, M. and Fairhead, J. (2011) Being 'with Medical Research Council': infant care and the social meanings of cohort membership in Gambia's plural therapeutic landscapes. In: Geissler, W. and Molyneaux, C. (eds.) *Evidence, Ethos and Experiment: The Anthropology and History of Medical Research in Africa*. Berghahn Books, Oxford, UK, pp. 77–98.

Molyneux, C. S., Peshu, N. et al. (2004) Understanding of informed consent in a low-income setting: three case studies from the Kenyan coast. *Social Science & Medicine* 59(12), 2547–2559.

O'Neill, O. (2003) Some limits of informed consent. *Journal of Medical Ethics* 29, 4–7.

MARTHA'S DILEMMA:

FOREIGN MEDICAL RESEARCH AS PUBLIC GOOD OR EXPLOITATION?

FACILITATOR'S NOTES

This story focuses on how medical research organizations may work to improve life and health in the future, but on the path towards realising this, they may not be contributing very much to people's lives and health in the here and now. This story asks you to put yourselves in the shoes of a research participant and consider her viewpoint. Even though participants in research projects may benefit from better care than in the public health system, this is only temporary and can create its own problems. Research organizations may be seen as both contributing to the public good, and at the same time building their privileged position on the very inequalities that they claim to alleviate. This case study aims to open up discussion on both the ethical and practical aspects of this paradox.

LEARNING OBJECTIVE

To recognise how and why participants may feel conflicted about the value of foreign-funded medical research, and that these differing views can co-exist and create dilemmas.

KEYWORDS

Inducements

Standards of care

Poverty

North-South relationships

Long-term engagement

MARTHA'S DILEMMA:
FOREIGN MEDICAL RESEARCH AS PUBLIC GOOD OR EXPLOITATION?

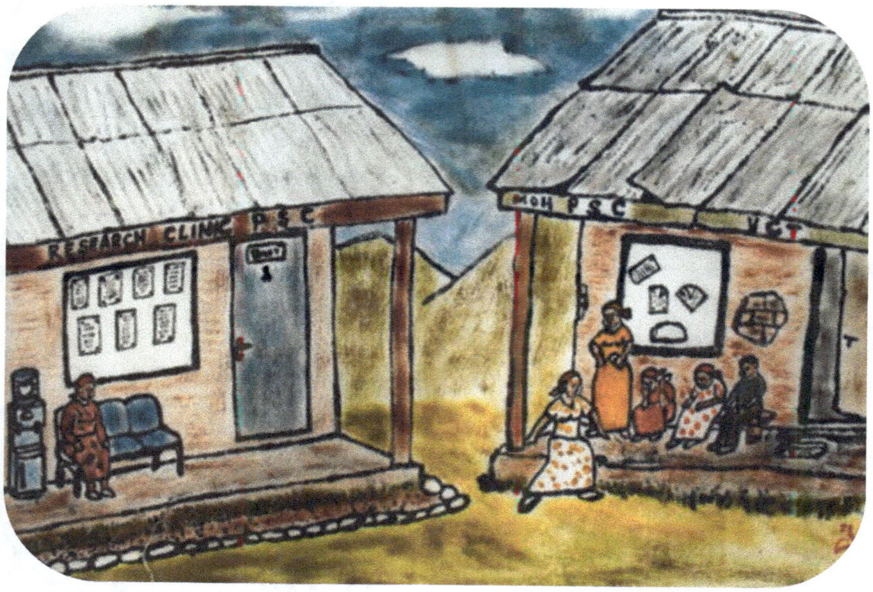

A RESEARCH CLASS SYSTEM

THE STORY

Martha is a well-educated woman in her early thirties. Some years back she had a formal job, but lost it because her company went bankrupt. Since then she has tried to run a small business as well as volunteering at a public health clinic, where she is much appreciated because of her skills and enthusiasm.

When pregnant with her third child, Martha gets involved with an internationally funded medical research project, which focuses on preventing mother-to-child HIV transmission via breastfeeding. This is not an easy decision for her. She thinks to herself: 'I don't like these researchers. Why are they testing us? Why aren't they doing it in their country? Is it because we are poor, or what?' She finds it hard to trust the motivations of the researchers.

At the same time, she understands that she will get first-rate care and advice regarding her child and her own health as long as she is involved with the project, which she would otherwise not be able to afford. She joins the research, and appreciates the knowledge she gains and the care that she and her infant receive.

After the project ends, Martha receives ongoing care at a public health clinic. Although she is always treated with respect at this free clinic, there are obvious differences between the resources available here and at the research project. She is quite upset about this difference. 'How can the researchers just come here and use us just because we are poor?' she thinks. 'It's an insult how their Principal Investigators get promotions because of us. They should not get an advantage out of our poverty. They are even contributing to it by giving us a little something in transport reimbursement, just to keep us quiet. They probably say behind our backs, "Africans are weak, just give them a bit of money and they'll do whatever you want." I don't know how the government permits them to come and do this work!'

Martha is unsure about whether to join the next research project when it opens for recruitment. She knows that certain research projects have to be carried out in Africa, because the particular conditions that the research aims to tackle are comparatively rare in Europe and the United States. Still, she finds it very odd that foreign-funded research organizations operate as almost independent entities in the overall healthcare system. She also feels that, although the medicines and treatments on trial are meant to benefit people like herself in the future, rich research organizations recruiting poor local people should do something further to improve their situation right away.

QUESTIONS

- Can you summarize Martha's ideas about foreign-funded medical research? What are the questions that are most important to her?
- What ideals do Martha's concerns express? Are these reasonable?
- Try listing the factors that would make Martha feel better about participating in the research. If Martha could see into the future, what would she hope to see coming out of the project?
- How about you? How much do you think research organizations should worry about improving people's lives and health here and now, as they carry out their exploration of how to improve the future?
- What about the past? What role do you think it plays when people are trying to understand present-day research?
- What practical problems might arise for the project, if concerns like Martha's are not addressed?

- Can you think of realistic ways in which a research project could try to draw links between present work, and the way it will be remembered in the future?

REFLECTION ON YOUR OWN EXPERIENCES

- Have you come across similar conflicting views of foreign-funded medical research? If so, how has your organization responded?

ACTIVITY

Split into groups of four to six people, depending on the size of your workshop, and discuss one of Martha's main areas of concern. Try to decide who is responsible for the problem, how it could be addressed, and how you could judge the outcome.

FURTHER READING

Crane, J.T. (2013) *Scrambling for Africa: AIDS, expertise, and the rise of American global health science*. Cornell University Press, Ithaca, New York.

Kingori, P. (2015) The 'empty choice': A sociological examination of choosing medical research participation in resource-limited sub-Saharan Africa. *Current Sociology* 63(5), 763–778.

Petryna, A. (2007) Clinical trials offshored: on private sector science and public health. *BioSocieties* 2(1), 21–40.

ROUTINE HEALTHCARE:
WHOSE OBLIGATION?

FACILITATOR'S NOTES

Clinical trials often provide free basic medical care for their participants. This is considered a benefit of participation, but also enables researchers to get the best possible data for their research. This story asks researchers to think about the full implications of providing 'routine' medical care for their participants. What are the limits of this provision? What do you do when the study can't, or won't, provide treatment for certain conditions, and your participants are unable to access it for themselves? Whose concern is the general health of research participants?

The story asks students to brainstorm best practice solutions to these kinds of situation. But it also invites them to think more widely and deeply about the underlying structures that create them. For example, one of the nurses in this story suggests that a participant is vulnerable, and thus unable to give reasonably informed consent, due to his poverty as well as his condition. Yet if this were true, who *would* be eligible to participate? Some critics do, in fact, argue that medical research is not ethical when it provides facilities that the national healthcare system does not. What does your group think about this?

In your discussion, you may want to ensure that you both touch on this wider debate, and also consider the elements of this specific case which make it difficult for the doctor in the story. Stigma and personal relationships also play a role. What similar experiences have your students had with research participants? How do their organizations support them through these dilemmas, or what solutions have they found?

LEARNING OBJECTIVE

To discuss best practice when providing routine medical care for trial participants, and to consider the limits of 'informed' consent

KEYWORDS

Research versus care

Poverty

Standards of care

Clinical responsibility

ROUTINE HEALTHCARE:
WHOSE OBLIGATION?

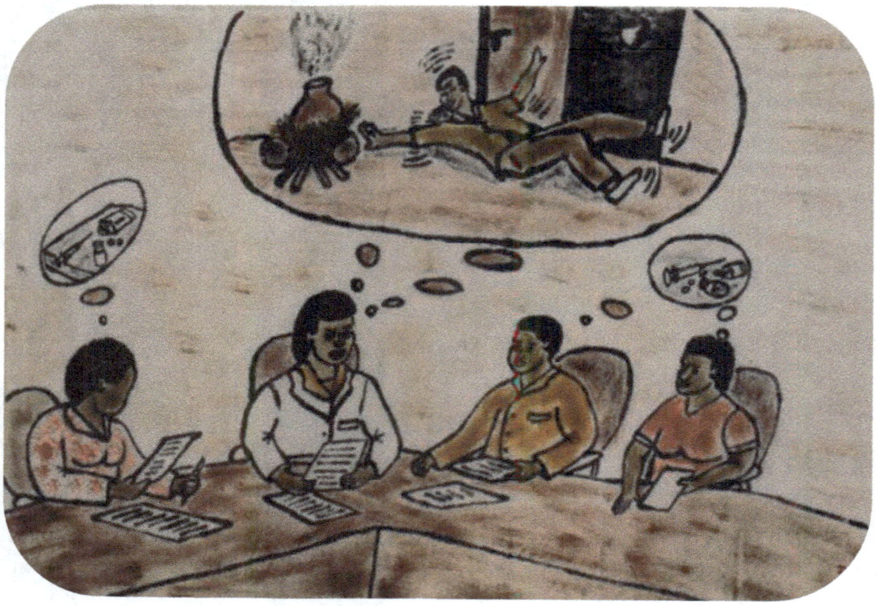

'WHAT CAN WE DO ABOUT THIS "AFFLICTION OF THE MOON"?'

THE STORY

Nwosa, a cook, decides to participate in a meningitis-related clinical trial, and is screened and enroled in it. He is required to live in the study area for two years, to follow a number of strict study procedures, and to make frequent visits to the clinic. Nwosa proves himself to be a very diligent participant. He always attends scheduled visits, and turns up unannounced for extra visits when sick.

During one of these extra visits one of the study doctors, Jane, begins to suspect that Nwosa has a serious medical condition which requires attention. She finds herself in a dilemma, and is unsure how best to assist him. She shares her suspicions about his condition with a senior colleague, but not with Nwosa, who is anyway treated for something else on this visit. Jane's colleague provides little guidance so she decides to just stick to the study and try to forget about her concerns for Nwosa's health beyond this.

However, during one of his next study visits Jane notices something unusual on his body: it looks like he has been burnt. She is curious, and asks him about it. Nwosa explains that he always falls down when the moon is up. He can't remember how he got burned, but thinks it was around that time. Jane's suspicion is confirmed: Nwosa, she now believes, has epilepsy. But it is not a condition she is experienced in. She does know that sufferers are often stigmatized in their community, and she is also aware that there is only one public specialist in the province, who is very difficult to see because he runs a busy and expensive private practice.

After this Jane decides to share her concerns at a team meeting. One of the nurses asks whether she has spoken to the Principal Investigator; as a study participant Nwosa is entitled to free routine medical care, so shouldn't this include treatment for epilepsy? 'I think it is your obligation as a doctor and as a researcher to make sure he gets treatment for his condition!' she says.

Jane replies that she has shared the issue with a senior colleague, but they were not helpful. But Nwosa's illness keeps bothering her. She says, 'Maybe I should find out what treatments and services are available at the local hospital.'

One of community interviewers asks Jane if there are any procedures in place to help staff decide what medical conditions qualify for 'routine care'. And what are the procedures for linking participants to outside care when services can't be provided by the study clinic? Jane cannot answer this question and promises to follow up on the issue.

The same community interviewer then adds, 'Nwosa is a vulnerable participant. He earns less than a dollar a day. He's extremely poor. He's only in the study because he knows he can come for those frequent sick visits. Should he even be in this study? How can he give informed consent?' 'Hmm,' says another doctor. 'If we categorize Nwosa as "vulnerable", then we should probably do the same with *all* our participants. Who will be left to participate?'

'But that's a totally different question! Poverty and epilepsy are not connected!' another member of staff responds. The meeting ends without any proper conclusions about how to assist the participant. The discussion about a specific case seems to have opened up a much wider uncertainty.

Time passes and Nwosa's next study visit comes around. This time, Jane finds he has more serious burns as a result of falling in the kitchen during his 'affliction of the moon'.

QUESTIONS

- ? Why do you think Jane does not share her suspicions with Nwosa?
- ? Why do you think she talks about his case in the team meeting? Why do you think it is a nurse who raises the question of Nwosa's general vulnerability? And why do you think the senior colleague was not very interested in the case?

- Why do you think Jane's specific question about what she should do leads to a wider discussion about involving poor people in medical research? What does this suggest about how the staff feel about their work in general?
- Do you think the senior colleague is supporting front-line staff enough? What might happen within the organization if nothing is done? What else could the organization do?
- What do you predict will happen to Nwosa if nothing is done? Why do you think decisions about his care are being postponed?
- What solutions for Nwosa's case can you come up with? What is the ideal solution? What is the most realistic solution?
- Do you agree with the community interviewer's classification of Nwosa as a 'vulnerable' participant? What factors do you think might be at play here? Should poor people be allowed to participate in trials, and if so, what measures should be put in place to ensure their consent is 'informed'?

REFLECTIONS ON YOUR OWN EXPERIENCES

- Does your study team have procedures and guidelines in place to help decide what qualifies as the free medical care you will offer to participants? How about referring participants on to other services? If so, what do you think about these documents? Could they be improved?
- Can you think of 'special' cases in your experience where you or a colleague has gone to extra lengths to provide extra medical care for a particular participant? Discuss these with the group and consider the ethics of this.
- How do you think an organization like Jane's can support its staff, in the face of working against widespread suffering (financial or medical)?

FURTHER READING

Mfutso-Bengo, J., Ndebele, P. et al (2008) Why do individuals agree to enrol in clinical trials? A qualitative study of health research participation in Blantyre, Malawai. *Malawai Medical Journal* 20. 37 - 41.

Whyte, S. R. (2014) Therapeutic research in low-income countries: studying trial communities. *Archives of Disease in Childhood* 99(11) 1029 -1032.

COMMUNITY AND FAMILY RELATIONSHIPS

TRAINING CASE STUDIES

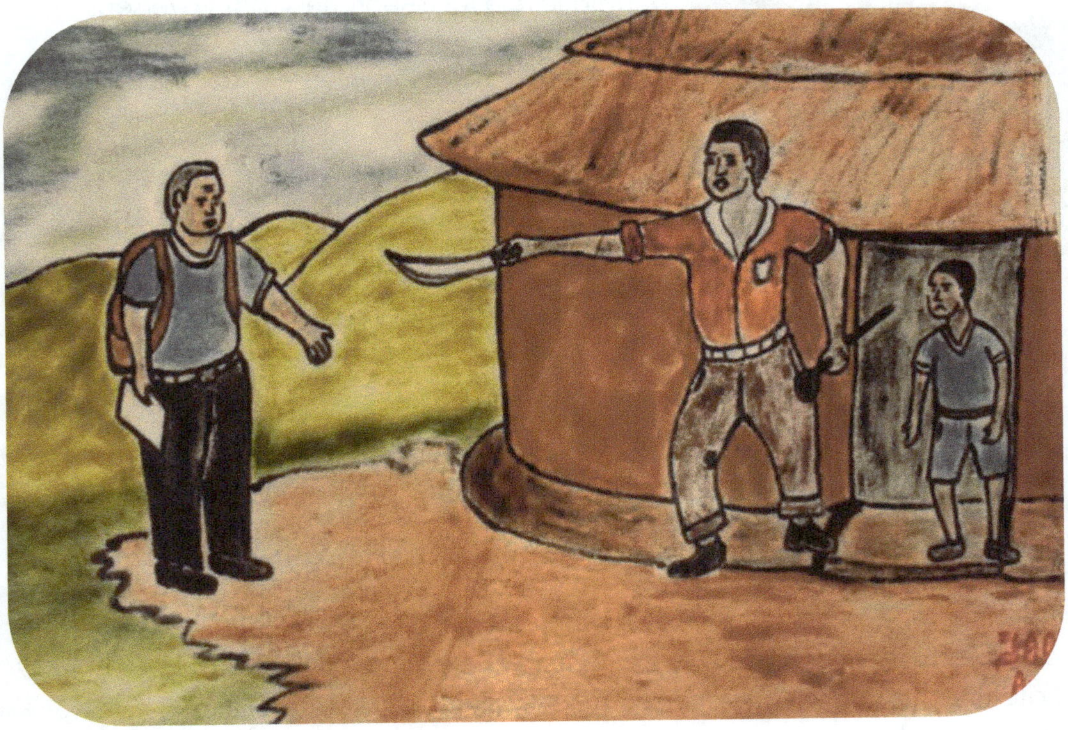

FRED FELT A LITTLE UNWELCOME WHEN HE CAME TO "CONSENT" GEORGE'S WIFE TO THE NEW STUDY...

COMMUNITY AND FAMILY RELATIONSHIPS

CASE STUDIES

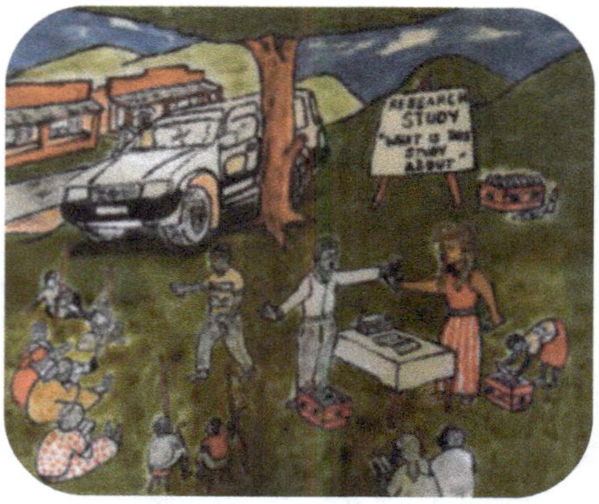

A COMMUNITY ENGAGEMENT MEETING

'Community engagement' is an increasingly important priority for research organizations and funders. Colonial medical research in Africa assumed a paternalistic, dogmatic role for researchers (both overseas and national), with communities cast as passive bodies to be studied and healed, in comparison with the more consultative role aimed for today. The concept of 'informed consent', let alone 'community consent', did not exist.

FURTHER READING

Geissler, P.W. and Pool, R. (2006) Editorial: Popular concerns about medical research projects in sub-Saharan Africa – a critical voice in debates about medical research ethics. *Tropical Medicine & International Health* 11(7), 975–982.

Angweniyi, V. et al. (2014) Complex realities: community engagement for a paediatric randomized controlled malaria vaccine trial in Kilifi, Kenya. *Trials* 15, 65.

Aellah, G. and Geissler, P.W (2016) Seeking Exposure: conversions of scientific knowledge in an African city. *Journal of Modern African Studies.*

Today global health researchers are exploring different permutations of community consultation and engagement. Some research stations set up community advisory boards or groups of elected representatives from different groups within communities. Others hold open community meetings to discuss, explain, and disseminate their research. Sometimes community members are invited to tour research stations, interview new researchers, and comment directly on protocols in their early stages.

Underlying these community engagement activities – and our collection of community relationships stories – are questions like: how do we best engage, work with and communicate our intentions and findings to different communities? How much involvement in research agenda setting and planning should – and can – communities actually have? Who 'owns' research? And what kind of meaningful understanding can there be between scientists and local communities, when the two groups sometimes see and experience the world differently?

An important aspect of community engagement involves understanding the ways power and authority operate in particular communities. Who has the authority to make decisions about research participation? To whom do individuals look to guide them? Religious leaders? Clan leaders? Opinion leaders? Local government? In many African contexts, decision-making is not necessarily done at an individual level. In response some research projects obtain consent for research participation from community leaders or household heads. What are the ramifications for this mode of consent for research and research ethics? What role does gender play in decision-making?

Another major concern in the relationship between researchers and communities is the destructive power of rumours about medical research. Rumours about blood and organ stealing, about birth control as a form of sterilization (including the association of bed-nets with infertility), and about the deliberate spreading of disease (for example through vaccines or holes in condoms) are common in sub-Saharan Africa. Rumours can have devastating effects on the success of projects and cause considerable anxiety for researchers. We agree that rumours need to be taken seriously and we have included several case studies on rumours here.

Our stories on rumour have the same underlying message: it is not particularly helpful to think about rumours in contrast to truth. Looking at rumours in this way makes them easy to dismiss as due to insufficient knowledge, or a lack of education or 'enlightened' modern thinking. However, as every researcher knows, simply increasing knowledge about the aims and practices of research in a community does not always lead to a reduction in rumour. This is because to understand rumours we need to look at them in the context of social relations, which are produced and changed by medical research. It is much more productive to think about rumour as a tool people use to express more nebulous anxieties about socio-economic conditions, and we need to take these anxieties seriously. Several of the case studies in this section explore this in more detail.

EVERYBODY'S CORRUPT:
UNDERSTANDING SUSPICION IN MEDICAL RESEARCH

FACILITATOR'S NOTES

This case is about a misunderstanding which arises when Community Advisory Board (CAB) members are paid their regular travel reimbursement in a different way after a meeting. CAB members suspect that the research staff are pocketing extra cash, and are not surprised by this, because they view corruption as common in all walks of life. In fact, what happened was not corruption but an administrative change which was not communicated effectively.

What is interesting about this case study is that when CAB members become aware of a change in routine procedures, they immediately suspect foul play. Prevailing corruption across different sectors of society feeds these suspicions, and instead of asking for an explanation, CAB members feel disappointed but not surprised. This case shows that sometimes the administrative requirements of research (in this case, to do with providing appropriate information according to set budgets) can be misinterpreted 'in the field' as reflecting something sinister, based on prior experiences of corruption. In your discussions you could focus on how these kinds of misinterpretations could be prevented, and also think about diverse understandings of travel reimbursements/sitting allowances.

You can also use this story as a jumping-off point to address more general issues of corruption in research which your group may have experienced. This story is about perceptions of corruption. But this could lead to a more general discussion of what corruption is. Encourage the group to discuss different

LEARNING OBJECTIVE

To reflect on situations where simple administrative practices in research may lead to suspicion in the community

KEYWORDS

Corruption

Community engagement

Money

Rumour

understandings of what corruption means, what forms 'real' corruption might take, who might be involved, the challenges involved in speaking about it, and what practices might offer the most effective safeguards in your specific research settings.

EVERYBODY'S CORRUPT:
UNDERSTANDING SUSPICION IN MEDICAL RESEARCH

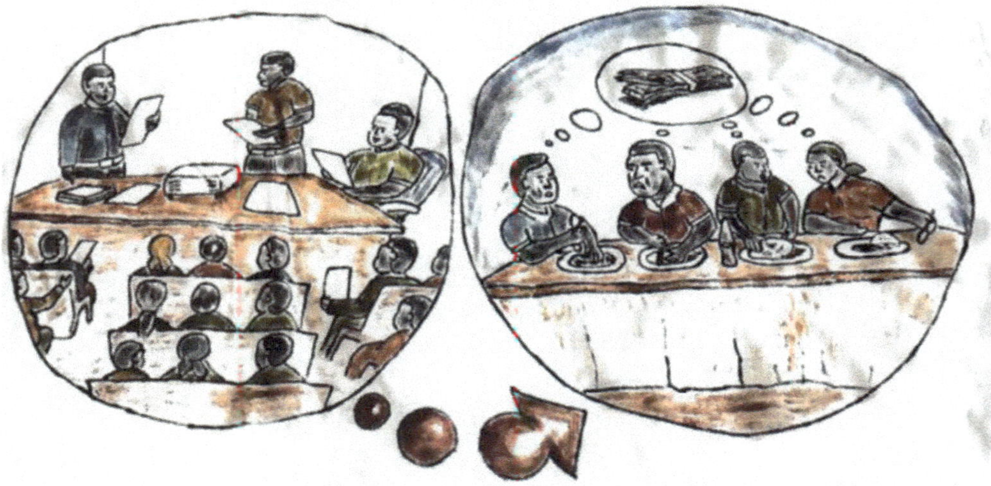

'THREE PROJECTS, BUT ONLY ONE LUNCH?!' COMMUNITY MEMBERS SUSPECT CORRUPTION

THE STORY

A large research station operating across several locations has established several Community Advisory Boards (CABs) to serve as community links and to test ideas for new studies. Today, one of the rural CABs is meeting to learn about three new studies. The 30 members sit in a meeting hall in the middle of their rural community, and three study coordinators give overviews of their proposed research using PowerPoint presentations. It's a very long morning, after which they all have lunch.

CAB members are usually given the equivalent of US$ 15 in cash per meeting, as compensation for their time and travel expenses. This is usually called 'transport reimbursement' or 'seating allowance'. To receive this allowance, they have to sign a designated sheet. Before ending the meeting, one of the study coordinators quickly explains that the three studies are related to each other, hence they decided to present at one meeting to save the busy CAB members having to come back three times. He tells them that because there are three studies represented today, they will divide the CAB into three groups for signing. He calls out their names and tells them which study coordinator they should go and see to sign for their allowance. There is a rumble of discontent amongst the group. This is a change from the normal routine. Why, they wonder, isn't everyone signing the same piece of paper? One of the CAB members notices that there are lots of blank lines under the ten names assigned to one of the studies.

During lunch the CAB members sit separately from the study coordinators. The members' conversation is all about this issue. They decide that the study coordinators must be corrupt. They speculate that each study was given money for the CAB meeting, but that the study coordinators got together and decided to only pay them the regular US$15 and pocket the rest, rather than pay them US$15 three times at three different meetings. That's what the blank lines are for – they are going to fill in fake names later. The study coordinators' bosses will never know what happened. The CAB members are annoyed, but not overly outraged. They don't tell the study coordinators their concerns directly. They are used to corruption; it's a normal occurrence. And anyway, they think the research organization is much less corrupt than the government.

QUESTIONS

- Can you untangle what is happening here? What are the key ethical issues?
- What specific factors do you think led to this situation?
- How is the time given by CAB members to fulfil their role valued by study coordinator and CAB members? Are there any notable differences in perspective? Why do you think this might be?
- What do you think about the way the study coordinators are administering the transport reimbursement on this occasion? How transparent were they being and what could they have done differently to avoid misunderstanding?
- Do you think the study coordinators and the CAB members share the same idea about what the transport reimbursement/sitting allowance money is for? Do you think it might represent something symbolic to CAB members? If so, and it seems that coordinators are stealing some of this money, what symbolic message might this send?
- What could have been done differently?
- What do you think the consequences of this situation might be? Is it 'just one of those things' which no one needs to worry too much about, or do you think it might have long-term consequences for this study or for future research?

THINKING ABOUT CORRUPTION MORE WIDELY

- What, in your opinion, is corruption? Are there other words and concepts related to it in your setting?

- ? What different forms can corruption (as the group has defined it) take in medical research?

- ? Who can be corrupt?

GROUP ACTIVITY

- ? Divide into small groups to discuss specific examples of ways in which 1-3 of the categories of people below could participate in research-related corruption, and report your discussions back to the others. For each category, provide a specific example and think about the motivation behind the person's actions. How might the corrupt person view their activities? Would they consider themselves corrupt? If not, why not?

    - Field-station Director
    - Overseas Principal Investigator
    - Study Coordinator
    - Drug company representative
    - Laboratory scientist
    - Auditor
    - Ethics Review Board member
    - Community fieldworker
    - Study pharmacist
    - Community Advisory Board member
    - Government minister
    - Human Resource manager
    - Administrator
    - Accountant/financial manager
    - Ministry of Health staff
    - Public hospital doctor
    - Local government official
    - Research participant

- ? What are some of the challenges in both recognizing and dealing with corruption?

- ? What practices could be put in place to help reduce corruption?

REFLECTION ON YOUR OWN EXPERIENCES

- Can you think of any similar situations to the one described in the story from your experience? How did you deal with them? Looking back now, what could you have done differently?
- Have you experienced any issues around corruption related to research activities? What kinds of corruption are there? How were they handled? What could have been done differently?

FURTHER READING

Newman, S.D., Andrews, J.O., Magwood, G.S. et al. (2011) Community advisory boards in community-based participatory research: a synthesis of best processes. *Preventing Chronic Disease* 8(3), A70.

Strauss, R.P., Sengupta, S., Quinn, S.C., Goeppinger, J., Spaulding, C., Kegeles, S.M., and Millett, G. (2001) The role of community advisory boards: involving communities in the informed consent process. *American Journal of Public Health* 91, 1938–1943.

BAD PRESS:
THE ORIGINS AND IMPACT OF 'BLOOD STEALING' RUMOURS

FACILITATOR'S NOTES

Stories and rumours about 'blood stealing' are found all over sub-Saharan Africa, and most researchers will encounter them at some point. This case study invites us to think critically about the origins of rumours about medical research. They can be a way to express dissatisfaction about broader issues, such as staff resentment and anger over inequality. It is important to recognise that concerns about blood have literal and symbolic meanings. People can be anxious about the amount of blood taken, and the pain involved, but the 'gift' of a highly valued substance also raises questions about fairness and exploitation. In this story, 'blood rumours' emerge as a way of expressing underlying complaints about access to jobs.

Rumours can also reflect social relationships. In this story, both the rumour itself, and the way the rumour ends up being reported in a newspaper, tell us something about different kinds of relationships. In discussions, you could encourage your students to think about what the rumour and how it is reported can teach us about the relationships between community members on the one hand, and both their leaders and the research station on the other. You may also want to discuss the role of the media, and think about how research programmes can work with media representatives.

Addressing rumours is not straightforward. It is not just a matter of trying to convince people that the facts of the rumour are wrong. The rumour itself may express deeper concerns about internationally funded medical research, how it operates, and what it aims to achieve, and mirror historical relationships between the country where the research is taking place and the countries of the international researchers.

LEARNING OBJECTIVE

To consider the origins and spread of rumours about medical research programmes, and to discuss how researchers could seek to manage these more proactively

KEYWORDS

Rumour

Media relations

Employment issues

Blood

BAD PRESS:

THE ORIGINS AND IMPACT OF 'BLOOD STEALING' RUMOURS

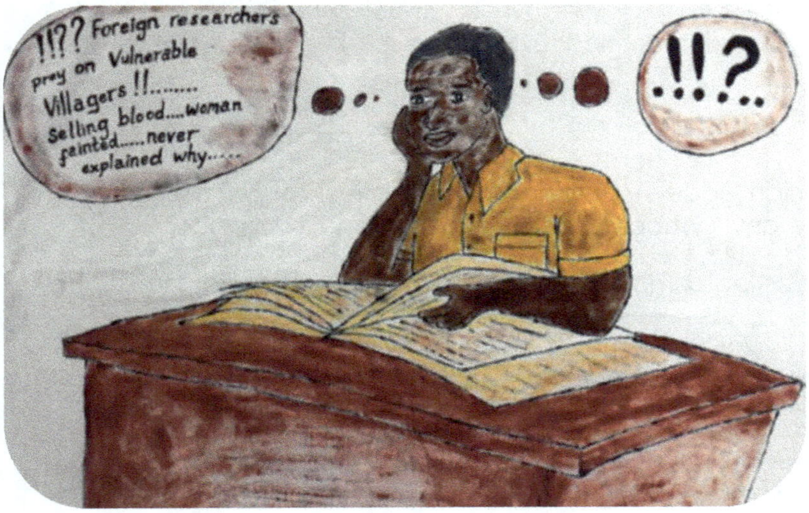
!!?? Foreign researchers prey on Vulnerable Villagers !!........ Selling blood....woman fainted......never explained why.....
.!!?..

'GOOGLING' HIS OWN NAME WAS NO LONGER FUN...

THE STORY

In this particular area, international medical research has been taking place for a long time, mostly without trouble. The research station employs a lot of people. Their rates of pay are the best in the region, and everyone competes for positions. Every time new jobs are advertised, a few people complain about corruption and tribal favouritism. After a while, these grumbles usually disappear.

This time, however, after a round of staff recruitment for a new vaccine trial, the Principal Investigator opens the national newspaper to find a special edition of 'The Reporter Investigates' focusing on his study. The article states that people are being experimented on by money-grabbing foreign researchers, who are taking advantage of their poverty to test new, dangerous drugs. Local 'opinion leaders' are quoted: '"Strangers regularly come to the villages and take our blood. They never tell us why. One widow even fainted after her blood was taken."'

The Principal Investigator is mentioned by name. Soon after putting down the newspaper his phone rings. It's his boss, calling from Vancouver. She wants to know how this could have happened.

The next week a corrective is published in the newspaper. In it, the director of the research station is quoted, explaining that the research station is run in partnership with the country's government, that all research is subject to approval by an ethics review board, that 90 per cent of the staff are local, and that the research station has a programme to disseminate findings. The damage is limited. But every time the Principal Investigator Googles his own name, the first link is a web forum discussion entitled 'Evil Western plot to sterilize our children'.

QUESTIONS

- Why do you think local opinion leaders were speaking negatively about the research? Do you think there might be any 'symbolic' truth in the story and if so, what?
- If you were the Principal Investigator, how would you answer your Canadian boss: how could this have happened?
- What are the potential long-term consequences of this media report, for the research programme, for the community, and for the Principal Investigator?
- What media strategies does your research organization have in place? Do you have any for social media? Who deals with media enquiries?
- Who are local opinion leaders you work with, and how should research organizations seek to work with them?

REFLECTION ON YOUR OWN EXPERIENCES

- Have you had any experience of rumours being reported on in the media? If yes, what happened and why do you think this happened? What did your organization try to do about this?
- Think about the types of rumours that are common in the areas where you work. What are they about, literally and symbolically? When do they usually surface, and how do you try to address them?
- How do rumours influence or affect the way you conduct research, engage with the local community, and recruit participants?

ACTIVITY

Split into small groups of four people and draft a media strategy for your research organization – or critically review your organization's current strategy. Think about how opinion leaders should be engaged. How, by whom, and in what type of forums? Why?

FURTHER READING

Mills, E. et al. (2005) Media reporting of tenofovir trials in Cambodia and Cameroon. *BMC International Health and Human Rights* 5(1), 6.

Singh, J.A. and Mills, E.J. (2005) The abandoned trials of pre-exposure prophylaxis for HIV: what went wrong? *PLoS Medicine* 2(9): e234.

Practical guides to engaging with the press can be found on Sci Dev Net website:

What journalists want from scientists and why:
http://www.scidev.net/global/communication/practical-guide/what-journalists-want-from-scientists-and-why.html (accessed 25 October 2015)

Explaining controversial issues to the media and the public:
http://www.scidev.net/global/communication/practical-guide/explaining-controversial-issues-to-the-media-and-t.html (accessed 25 October 2015)

How do I become media savvy? http://www.scidev.net/global/communication/practical-guide/how-do-i-become-media-savvy-.html?from=related%20articles (accessed 25 October 2015)

PEOPLE WILL ALWAYS TALK:

PROTECTING PARTICIPANTS FROM STIGMA IN AN HIV STUDY

FACILITATOR'S NOTES

In many parts of Africa, HIV-related stigma, is still very real, and in some places simply being associated with transnational research represents a risk of being stigmatized as HIV positive. This case study follows a microbicide trial and the efforts study staff make to limit gossip about participants' HIV status. It asks how much responsibility staff can and should have to try to control what people are saying about participants, especially when participants belong to a group considered 'at risk'.

The case provides a powerful example of the way medical and social issues can become entangled. The researchers in the story put in a lot of effort to protect their participants. However, we invite you to think about how effective their solution really was, or whether it could have had other negative consequences. You may want to explore other possible approaches, for example, sharing information about the study with the general public to emphasize that it focuses on women who do not (yet) have HIV. Going further, the case raises the question if researchers' efforts to protect their participants could be contributing to stigma. You might also want to discuss whether the changing nature of the HIV epidemic altered the way people view HIV? If yes, does this mean we can/should change the way we think about stigma in relation to medical research? You may be able to draw links with ethical arguments made for opt-out or provider-initiated HIV testing, which have suggested that giving HIV testing a special status of 'voluntary' has actually contributed to stigma (see further reading).

LEARNING OBJECTIVE

To reflect on some of the social and economic problems associated with researching HIV among 'at risk' communities, and to consider how far and in what ways researchers on this type of project are responsible for addressing these issues

KEYWORDS

Rumour

Confidentiality

Home visits

Stigma

PEOPLE WILL ALWAYS TALK:
PROTECTING PARTICIPANTS FROM STIGMA IN AN HIV STUDY

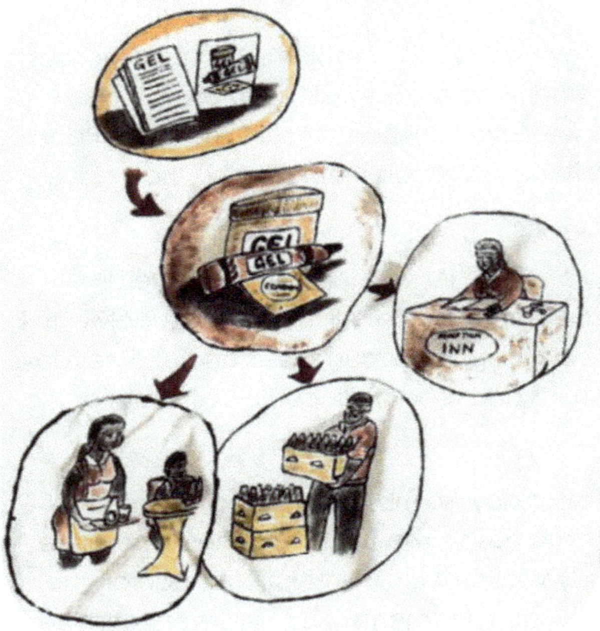

JACINTA WORRIED THAT HER CUSTOMERS WOULD THINK SHE HAD HIV IF SHE PARTICIPATED IN THE STUDY

THE STORY

Jacinta works in a bar. One night she is approached at work by a smartly dressed lady who hands her a leaflet about a study, and invites her to attend a meeting the next day in a community hall to find out more. Jacinta has heard from other girls that research studies are a good way to get free healthcare, so she goes along.

At the meeting, the study coordinator, Dr Agava, explains the project to the 20 women who have gathered. She tells them that the trial aims to find out whether a microbicide gel will protect women from HIV infection, and that researchers are looking for HIV negative women to take part. Participants will be asked to use the gel every time they have sex, and to attend the local government HIV clinic regularly, where study doctors working alongside government medical personnel will test them for HIV and other STIs. The doctors will also distribute more gel and administer questionnaires about participants' sexual behaviour. If participants miss appointments, they may receive follow-up visits at home. They will also receive money for their transport and time, as well as free healthcare throughout the 12-month study.

Most of the women are enthusiastic. Jacinta likes the idea of the gel; if it works, it will be helpful, as most of her boyfriends don't want to use condoms. But she is worried about visiting the HIV clinic regularly. The study coordinator asks the women for their thoughts about the study. Jacinta puts up her hand and says: 'The problem is that this is a small city. If people see me going to the clinic every month, they will talk. Everyone will think I have HIV. Then people will gossip about me. It will give me stress.'

Dr Agava asks the women for suggestions about how to solve this problem. Jacinta proposes they hold the clinic in a secret place. One of the other women suggests using one of the rooms in a local guesthouse. 'People will just think we have "business" there,' she says. 'People already think that I am a parking lady [prostitute]. Better that than them thinking that I have HIV'.

As a result of this discussion, the researchers set up a 'clinic' for women to visit in several guesthouses on different days of the week. They are careful not to talk about this widely in the community, and the guesthouses continue to provide services for customers on the other days of the week. Everyday activities, such as small markets and food stalls, continue in front of the guesthouses during clinics.

One day Jacinta is asked to work on her allotted clinic day, so misses her appointment. The next day one of the study staff visits her house. Jacinta has shown the researchers where she lives. David, one of the field staff, comes in the study vehicle, with its institutional logo on the side. Jacinta lives in a large compound with lots of small apartments, and his driver parks the vehicle inside the gate because, in this neighbourhood, he doesn't want to risk leaving it outside.

David is worried about the home visit, fearing that after this Jacinta might not want to continue with the study. He apologizes to Jacinta for bringing the vehicle. 'But,' he tells her, 'I can't take your samples back to our lab on public transport, so I couldn't come in secret. I hope this visit doesn't cause problems for you with your neighbours.'

He is surprised when Jacinta replies, nonchalantly, 'Oh, don't worry about that. People will always talk. People already whisper, "Oh, you know that lady in the bar? She's in that study for ladies who are sick." But just ignore them. If you don't listen to people like that they will talk for two or three days then they will stop. And if they talk loudly I just tell them they are ignorant and wrong.'

'Oh, OK, that's good,' says David, thinking, 'Huh, this is a strong lady.'

QUESTIONS

- What are key ethical issues at stake in this situation? Do you think participants are being oversensitive about their 'reputations'? What else do you think might be behind Jacinta's 'stress'?
- What responsibility do you think the study coordinator has to ensure that participants are not exposed to stigma? What responsibility do the women themselves have?
- Why might Jacinta have been so relaxed about David's visit? Were you surprised at her response? Even if researchers do their very best to protect participants, how far do you think they really can control how their work is perceived?
- What do you think about the decision to run clinics in the guesthouses instead of at the hospital? Could this have compromised the women's reputations in other ways? (Remember that the government clinic is known to provide HIV testing, as well as treatment.) Could there be other consequences to removing the clinics from the government clinics, in terms of the relationship between the researchers and the government?
- How else could the field staff have tried to mitigate rumours?
- What underlying messages about HIV might the focus on secrecy have sent out to the women, and to the wider community?

REFLECTION ON YOUR OWN EXPERIENCES

- Can you think of similar situations from your experience where you may have tried, and struggled, to engage with the ways your work has been perceived?
- Looking back at this, do you have any ideas of what could you have done differently?

FURTHER READING

April, M. (2010) Rethinking HIV exceptionalism: the ethics of opt-out HIV testing in sub-Saharan Africa. *Bulletin of the World Health Organization* 88, 703–708. DOI: 10.2471/BLT.09.073049 Available at: http://www.who.int/bulletin/volumes/88/9/09-073049/en/ (accessed 25 October 2015).

Stangl, A.L. and Grossoman, C.I. (Eds.) (2013) Global action to reduce HIV stigma and discrimination. *Journal of the International Aids Society*, Volume 16, Supplement 2. Available at: http://www.jiasociety.org/index.php/jias/issue/view/1464 (accessed 25 October 2015). Includes webinar.

LOST IN TRANSLATION:
PUBLIC COMMUNICATION AND POWER RELATIONS

FACILITATOR'S NOTES

This case is about community engagement in research – specifically, initial community entry. It aims to help think through the role, remit and constitution of representative public bodies in health research. The story describes what happens when a research team goes about setting up a community advisory board (CAB): the team's disagreements become evident in public meetings, there are questions over how representative the CAB is likely to be, and governmental administrative leaders are keen to secure leadership within it. The case draws attention to the critical importance of internal work relationships, communication, and trust among research staff, and also the need for a unified, coherent approach in order to establish good relationships with the local community. It also invites reflection on the role of gender relations and power in this process.

In your discussions about the story, please note that getting this kind of community entry right can be very difficult. Conditions are never perfect. Some issues to draw out might include the fact that, while community members clearly valued the trial coordinator's presence, it would probably have been better if she had allowed the community relations officer to deliver the agreed message in the local language. This would have facilitated comprehension and improved team dynamics. It would also be a good idea for these two colleagues to discuss who should be responsible for the coordination of the CAB. Then, as the CAB starts, it will also be essential to think about its role, and whether it will run autonomously or with support from the main research unit.

LEARNING OBJECTIVE

To explore best practices and challenges in initiating community entry and creating community advisory boards, and to reflect on the importance of staff unity when engaging with the community

KEYWORDS

Community entry

Community engagement

Gender

Translation

LOST IN TRANSLATION:

PUBLIC COMMUNICATION AND POWER RELATIONS

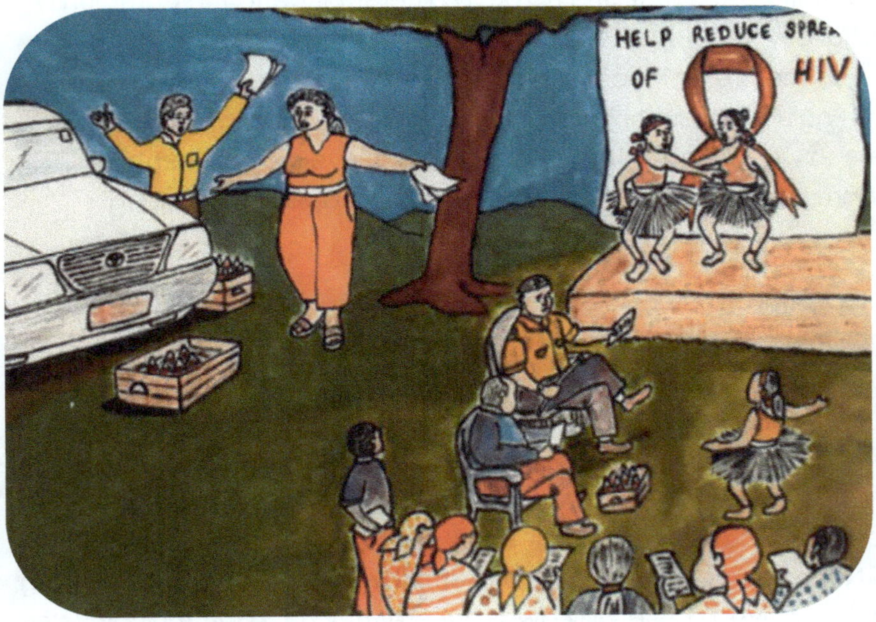

WHILE THE CHILDREN DANCED FOR THE GUESTS, NOAH AND EMZARA PROVIDED THE REAL ENTERTAINMENT

THE STORY

At a transnational research station in central Africa, preparations are underway for an exciting multi-sited trial of a new HIV prevention tool. The research station has been chosen as one of the first sites for this hotly anticipated project, which is bringing a lot of funding and prestige – as well as pressure – to the station and staff.

The trial participants will be recruited from public health facilities in a rural area, which has not previously been involved in any research activities. To prepare the community, the research team decide they need to establish a Community Advisory Board (CAB). The male, American trial manager, Ham, the young female African coordinator, Emzara, and the research station's African community relations officer, Noah, draw up plans for this.

They start by visiting local government officers to explain the purpose of the trial and their reasons for setting up a CAB. They tell the officers that they would like community members to nominate potential CAB members during the officers' regular 'barazas' – a grassroots vehicle for discussion of community concerns, solving disputes between neighbours, and communicating administrative and political measures and regulations. NGOs and other organizations often use barazas to introduce themselves and their projects to the community. The officers agree to this and they set dates for the team's attendance.

Before the first baraza Ham, Emzara and Noah prepare a script to explain what the trial is about, why they want to set up CAB, and how the nomination process will work. Emzara, the trial coordinator, is a young, ambitious scientist. She is from a different tribe to the community, and is originally from the capital city, but has been learning some of the local tribal language in preparation. She plans to start the presentation with an introduction in the local language, but will then have to revert to English, with Noah, the community liaison officer, translating. Noah is in his late fifties. Before this job he had a long career in mid-level government administration. He was also born in this area, so he can speak and understand the local language in its full complexity.

On the day of the meeting Ham, Emzara and Noah set off early in a Toyota 4x4, but by the time they arrive at the baraza, scheduled for 11am, the government officer has assembled over 50 community members and the meeting is already in full swing. The government officer and his assistants, dressed in full uniform, stop the meeting to greet the research team at their vehicle and lead them to the front of the gathering, where people are sitting in a circle under a group of trees. Younger women, especially those with children, sit on the grass on pieces of cloth to protect their clothes; older women sit amongst the older men on chairs and benches in a half-circle behind them. Not many young men are present; fewer than ten stand, listening and chatting quietly among themselves, a little way away, where they have left their bicycles and motorbikes in the background.

Ham, the foreign visitor, is given the only spare chair, next to the government officer at the front. Emzara and Noah stand next to them while the government officer introduces the three of them in turn. Then Emzara steps forward to greet the gathering in the local language. This breaks the ice and the ambience remains positive when Emzara reverts to English to communicate the scripted information. Emzara reads separate portions of the text and, as agreed, Noah translates in turn. Halfway through, Emzara notices that Noah has gone ahead of her in his translation. But she is not sure what he is saying. This results in some tension among the staff, which is not immediately visible to the gathering.

At the end of their script, the government officer helps Emzara and Noah to explain how the nomination process will work. Attendees are separated into various groupings – women's groups, church groups, and village elders – who are asked to come up with two names amongst themselves for CAB nominees from their group. After this, the nominees' names are read out to the larger gathering, to resounding applause. The nominees pass their details to Emzara and Noah, who tell them they will be in contact to arrange a time to meet up individually for a separate selection process.

The research team have now finished what they came to the meeting to do, and want to leave, as it looks like the baraza could continue all day. The government officer, however, has other ideas. He has organized for some primary school children to give a dramatic dance performance on HIV to the research team. The children are dressed in their dance outfits, and look very disappointed when it seems the team will leave. Ham tells the group that of course he would love to watch the show. He motions to Emzara and Noah that they can withdraw and carry on with their work by the vehicle. They have lots of phone calls to make, so they move away from the gathering and the children begin their performance.

Over by the vehicle, Emzara and Noah start talking about the translation issue. Emzara is upset. She tells Noah it is not just about usurping the predefined format, but it is also about gender. She thinks that, given the nature of the HIV prevention tool being trialled, young women's collaboration is key, hence the lead should be taken by a woman and not a man in public meetings. She also suggests that she should chair the CAB, as the female African member of the team. Emzara and Noah are now talking quite loudly in fast English. Some members of the gathering have started to look over at them. Ham pretends he can't hear them and smiles at the performers.

Later that day, Noah receives a call from the chief government officer, volunteering himself as chair of the CAB.

QUESTIONS

- Why do Ham, Emzara and Noah write a script for the baraza? Was this a good idea?
- Why do you think they decided to use both the local language and English to explain the proposed trial and plans for the CAB?
- Why do you think Noah may have started to translate ahead of Emzara?
- What can be done to promote good working relations and trust in multi-disciplinary, multi-ethnic, and international research teams?
- Was the baraza the best place to launch the project? Are all members of the community equally involved in it, and does this matter for the CAB and the trial?
- What do you think about the nomination process the research team chose to identify potential CAB members? What was good about this, and what could have been done better?
- Do you think the nominees will have understood that nomination did not necessarily mean that they would become CAB members?
- What do you think about Emzara's suggestion that a female African member of the research team should assume responsibility for coordinating the CAB?

- ? What do you think about the government officer's request to be chair of the CAB? How should the research team respond to this? Do you think the team's behaviour at the baraza had a role in his suggestion?

REFLECTION ON YOUR OWN EXPERIENCES

- ? Does this case remind you of any of your own experiences? What was happening, and what did you do? What could you have done differently?
- ? Do you have a CAB at your workplace? If so, how was this set up, and how does it function? Who do you think should select CAB members?
- ? What role do you think CAB members should play? What is a CAB's mandate?
- ? What do you think about the relationship between researchers and CAB members?

ACTIVITY

Split the group up into groups of four to six, and ask them to think through how they would set up a community advisory board or a similar representative body. If you already have such bodies at your workplace, you could ask the groups to review current practice and come up with ideas of how they could be improved. You could get groups to:

- critically review any existing guidelines (e.g. nomination processes, the mandate of community representatives, the role of the research team);
- report on their experiences of interacting with community representatives;
- discuss the value of such representative bodies.

FURTHER READING

Diallo, D.A., Doumbo, O.K., Plowe, C.V., Wellems, T.E., Emanuel, E.J., and Hurst, S.A. (2005) Community permission for medical research in developing countries. *Clinical Infectious Diseases* 41, 255–259.

Marsh, V., Kamuya, D., Rowa, Y., Gikonyo, C., and Molyneux, S. (2008) Beginning community engagement at a busy biomedical research programme: experiences from the KEMRI CGMRC-Wellcome Trust Research Programme, Kilifi, Kenya. *Social Science and Medicine* 67, 721–733.

HUSBAND OUT OF TOWN:

GENDER RELATIONS AND DECISION-MAKING

FACILITATOR'S NOTES

This case explores how children are recruited for trials, how parents are involved, and the role of gender relations in this kind of research. In the story, a first-time mother provides consent for her infant to take part in a vaccine trial without her husband's involvement, with unfortunate consequences. The case raises key questions around participants' motivation for enrolment in trials; communication and comprehension around participation; how much time is given to participants to make decisions, and in what conditions; and whether and how consent could involve people more fairly.

One could argue that the mother in the story should have been given more time to think about joining the research. She could have been given information materials to take home, to help her talk to her husband and other family members about the project. Her husband could have signed a form at home for her to take into the clinic, to show they both agree. The problem with this is that it places the burden of communication on the mother, requires the father to be present and willing to engage, and makes certain assumptions about gender relations and power. It is therefore important that researchers think more creatively about how they can engage effectively with both parents.

Before the session it would be a good idea to review how your institute organizes trial recruitment and parental consent on behalf of minors. You might also want to check what the legal requirements are in your context.

LEARNING OBJECTIVE

To reflect upon the informed consent process, especially in relation to involving both parents of children involved in trials in decision-making

KEYWORDS

Gender

Informed consent

Minors consent

Partner involvement

HUSBAND OUT OF TOWN:
DECISION-MAKING AND GENDER RELATIONS

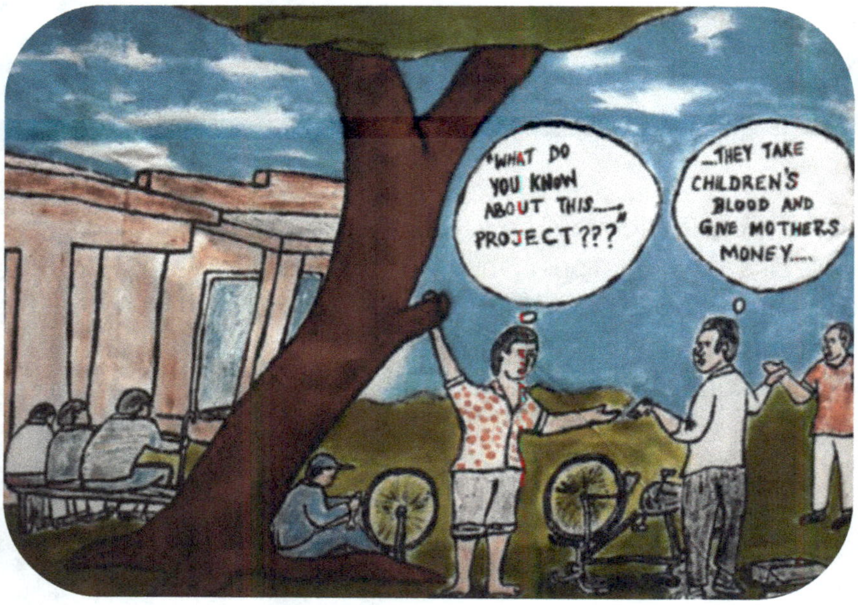
"WHAT DO YOU KNOW ABOUT THIS..... PROJECT???"
...THEY TAKE CHILDREN'S BLOOD AND GIVE MOTHERS MONEY.....

DAVID FIRST LEARNT ABOUT THE RESEARCH PROJECT FROM HIS FRIENDS

THE STORY

Grace, a 20-year-old first-time mum, lives with her husband's family in a village which has limited access to public transport. She is worried that her five-week old baby Nathan is not putting on weight, so she decides to take him to the health clinic in town to have him checked and weighed. On her 30-minute walk to the clinic she meets her friend Anna, whose baby is about the same age. Anna has just come from the clinic, and starts telling Grace all about a new project that she has just joined. She is full of praise: the nurses are friendly, a doctor checked her baby, and they will be vaccinating him against meningitis. They took great care of her baby, and even gave her some money (the equivalent of US$5) to help her pay for transport even though she usually walks. She is going to use the cash to add some meat to the stew she is preparing tonight. Grace wonders if she can join this project as well. Anna tells her to go to the side buildings next to the main clinic and talk to the nurses there.

When Grace arrives at the clinic she sees other mothers with young children sat on benches outside the side buildings. She makes her way over and sits down with them. They greet her and they all start talking about what they have heard about the project. A nurse comes out and gives everyone a letter to read, saying that she will go over what is written in the letter with them all in about five minutes. Nathan has woken up and needs to be breastfed, so Grace settles him while she waits for the nurse to return. She reads the first couple of paragraphs of the five-page letter.

The nurse returns, sits down on a chair in front of the mothers, and explains that the main purpose of the project is to test whether a new meningitis vaccine works. She then starts to read out the letter, getting some of the mothers to take turns in reading certain sections out loud. She stops regularly to encourage them to ask questions and interact. It takes almost 30 minutes to finish reading the letter, by which time Grace is getting tired and hungry. She is happy that she was not asked to read aloud, but feels she has not really understood everything the nurse explained. It seems to be some sort of aid project, and she is keen for Nathan to be checked by the project doctor before she goes home, so she decides to enrol him. The nurse asks Grace whether she needs to talk to Nathan's father before she signs the consent form. Grace tells the nurse that Nathan's father works and lives away from home during the week, and she can't contact him because she has run out of mobile phone credit. She does not think he will mind, so she goes ahead and signs the consent form.

The nurses then weigh Nathan, and the doctor does a full assessment. Grace is really impressed by the doctor, who examines the child thoroughly, undressing him and palpating his abdomen. She is relieved when he tells her that Nathan is in good health. She gets a bit upset when the nurses and doctors take a blood sample, but feels better when they give her a cup of tea. Over tea, the mothers share their experience with the caring staff, and appreciate their hospitality. Before Grace leaves she is given the transport money Anna told her about, and is asked to come back in a week's time for Nathan's first course of vaccines.

When she arrives home Grace has to start preparing the evening meal straightaway. She completely forgets to tell anyone about the project. Even when her husband, David, comes home for the weekend, she does not remember. It is only when he has left again that she recalls that she meant to tell him about the project, but then she thinks to herself: 'It is not worth bothering him, he relies on me to take care of little Nathan, and anyway he might just want me to give him the transport money.'

A few weeks later Grace forgets one of her project appointments – it is harvest time and she has gone to market to sell maize. Her husband has come home to help with the harvest, and is at home when a project fieldworker arrives on his motorbike. The fieldworker has come to check whether Grace and Nathan are OK, and to remind them to come to the clinic. David is surprised to see a young man making his way into their compound, and asks why he has come. The fieldworker explains that he works for the meningitis project and needs to check up on Nathan. David is angry that this man seems to be on familiar terms with his wife and son, and chases him away. He then gets on his bike and makes his way to the local shops to talk to some of his friends about it. He finds a group of men sitting together under a tree and quizzes them about what they know about the programme.

They tell him that they have heard that it involves researchers testing children and sending their blood overseas, and that the researchers give the mothers money. David returns home even more concerned, and when Grace gets back from the market he demands that she take Nathan out of the programme straight away. Grace tries to explain what the project is about and how well Nathan is being looked after, but her own understanding of the research is limited, and David does not want to listen. He is really angry so Grace sends a message to the project team, explaining that Nathan will not be able to continue to participate.

QUESTIONS

- Is David just being 'backward' or a dominant man? What effect has the project had on his relationship with Grace?
- How could this situation have been avoided? If Grace had been given information and a form home for her husband to sign, what would have been the benefits and disadvantages? What would this suggest about the balance of power and responsibility in their relationship?
- What should the research team do when they receive Grace's message?
- How much time do parents need to be given before deciding about whether to enrol their children in research? What else might have made Grace rush into agreeing?
- Do both parents play the same role? Do projects need to gain both parents' consent, and if so, must this be done in the same way? What might this mean for project planning?
- Is information and knowledge in this situation the only key to satisfactory consent?
- Could both Grace and David's confusion have been avoided? If yes, what do you think could have been done by the research staff?

REFLECTION ON YOUR OWN EXPERIENCES

- Have you come across similar situations? How have you dealt with them?

ACTIVITY

Get into groups of three to four and draft a recruitment strategy for a children's trial, involving both mothers and fathers in a way that seems appropriate. Think about the legal requirements of consent as well as international ethical guidelines and national laws.

FURTHER READING

Mathews, C., Guttmacher, S.J., Flisher, A.J., Mtshizana, Y., Hani, A., Zwarenstein, M. (2005) Written parental consent in school-based HIV/AIDS prevention research. *American Journal of Public Health*, 95(7), 1266–1269.

Pace, C., Talisuna, A., Wendler, D. et al. (2005) Quality of parental consent in a Ugandan malaria study. *American Journal of Public Health* 95(7), 1184–1189.

CHOP YOUR MONEY!: CHALLENGES IN RECRUITMENT AND ENFORCING STUDY RULES

FACILITATOR'S NOTES

This case study explores the role of both community and family relationships in recruiting and retaining participants. Medical research institutions employ several strategies to recruit and retain trial participants, often making use of informal structures such as Community Advisory Boards, peer leaders, or community liaison personnel to try to reach their target community. However, despite these efforts, smooth relationships with participants are not guaranteed, and recruiting and retaining people remains a challenge. This case study invites us to think critically about questions related to the recruitment and retention of trial participants. It provides an example of the requirement for female participants to use contraception in a trial, and the impossibility of 'enforcing' this. It invites you to think about the role of male partners in decision-making about following study rules.

It also raises questions over the role of reimbursements in the recruitment process. Attempts to control the problems could infringe on participants' basic rights. The study also points to the underlying suspicion and cynicism with which communities can view trials, and the difficulties Community Advisory Board members face in trying to overcome this mistrust.

None of these questions are straightforward, so you will need to take care in how you manage the ensuing discussions.

LEARNING OBJECTIVE

To consider challenges in recruiting participants and ensuring they follow study rules

KEYWORDS

Informed consent

Gender

Money

Recruitment

Partner involvement

CHOP YOUR MONEY!:

CHALLENGES IN RECRUITMENT AND ENFORCING STUDY RULES

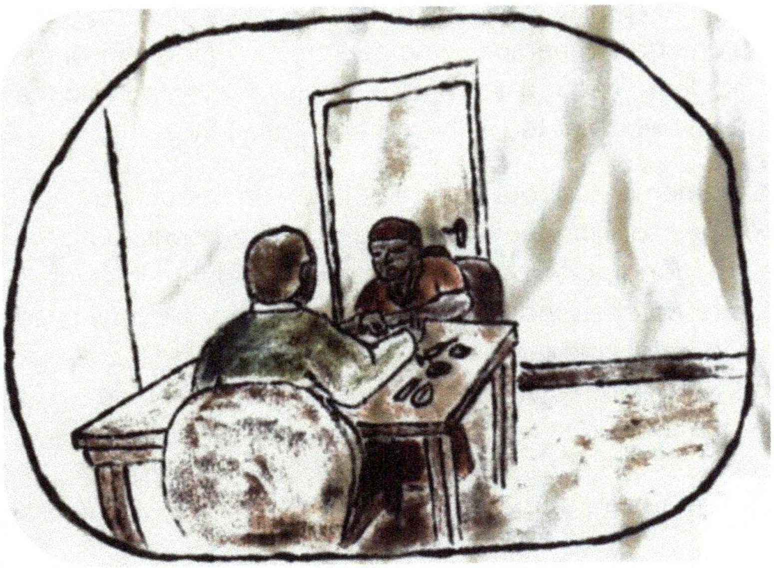

'DON'T WORRY, I'LL PRACTICE ABSTINENCE DURING THE TRIAL,' SAID MARY, REJECTING THE OFFER OF CONTRACEPTIVES. 'UM... OK...' SAID THE DOCTOR DOUBTFULLY

THE STORY

A story in a major national newspaper quotes a group of scientists from the National AIDS Vaccine Institute, expressing their frustration with the high pregnancy rates among women participating in vaccine trials. All women are advised not to become pregnant during the trials, due to the unknown side effects of the vaccine, however in one study a number of women conceived children. They have apparently been coerced by their partners to have unprotected sex.

All the women in the trial have had the risks explained to them, and were offered a choice of contraception for free. Those who became pregnant were the ones who opted for abstinence as their preferred method of contraception, so in the article the scientists recommended that abstinence should no longer be an option given to trial participants. They state, 'Every effort must be made to ensure that trial participants do not get pregnant during the specified periods, and that they are retained until the end of the vaccine trial.'

After reading the newspaper article, Community Advisory Board (CAB) members in the National Aids Vaccine institute start talking about some of the frustrations they experience in participant recruitment. Many of the members were trial participants themselves before joining the board. Researchers hoped this would help with recruitment, as they hoped that ex-participants could allay fears among community members and use their experience to convince others to join the vaccine trials.

According to CAB members, however, this is never enough to convince suspicious community members. 'Any time we tell them that we have participated in a previous study, they do not believe us. They say we are lying,' says one board member. Another remarks: 'I took part in a trial with other community members, but they were not convinced that I was injected with the same vaccine as they were. They thought I was injected with a different substance.'

When the researchers talked to the CAB members about the issue of women becoming pregnant during the trial, the CAB members said that perhaps these girls didn't participate for the right reasons and therefore were not 'good participants'. They pointed out that this was part of a bigger problem. They told the researchers that they thought many people they try to recruit take advantage of the process to obtain money, with no intention of ever participating. Some of the participants who refuse to enrol only at the final stages of the recruitment process tell CAB members that this is due to fear of the vaccine, yet, the CAB members argue, they seem very keen to complete the initial counselling and screening sessions to obtain the transport reimbursements for these sessions.

One of the CAB members explains: 'You know, in the recruitment we often recruit our friends. Some of them have been quite frank and told us: "We knew all along that we would not take part in the trials, but you guys pay lots of money for transport, and give us snacks any time we come. We just wanted to chop your money." Perhaps those women who conceived were just thinking about chopping money and ignored the rules of the research.' (This expression, 'to chop money', is coined from a popular African song and means 'taking someone's money without giving anything in return'.)

'But on the other hand,' one of the male CAB members says, 'we all know that pregnancy is an issue between men and women, not between women and researchers! Perhaps these ladies did not tell their husbands about the trial.'

QUESTIONS

- Do you think the female trial participants 'intended' to get pregnant despite enrolling? What are the problems with this concept of 'intention' in this sort of case? What does this tell us about informed consent?
- What do you think about the scientists' suggestion that trial participants must use contraception methods other than abstinence to ensure that they do not get pregnant? What about those whose relationship status changes during a trial or before a trial, and who therefore decide they want to have children? What about participants or potential participants whose health or personal circumstances make it difficult for them to use contraceptive methods consistently?
- Do you think there was a need to involve participants' male partners more in the trial? How could this be achieved?
- Given the problems of recruitment, what ethical issues emerge from the use of financial inducements to recruit trial participants – for the trial, and for the potential participants?
- Can you think of any reasons why the friends of the CAB members, who were recruited to the trials, were very opportunistic about trying to 'chop' the money?
- What do the quotes in this story tell us about the experiences of Community Advisory Board members? Do you think the researchers could do more to support them, and if so, how?

REFLECTION ON YOUR OWN EXPERIENCES

- Have you observed similar opportunism when it comes to getting a share of research resources – maybe even before participants take part? If, yes, what happened, and how did you deal with this?
- What is your view about the role of CAB members or similar representatives? Should they be actively involved in recruitment activities?

FURTHER READING

Geissler, W. (2011) 'Transport to where?': reflections on the problem of value and time *à propos* an awkward practice in medical research. *Journal of Cultural Economy* 4(1), 45–64.

Painter, M.T., Kassamba, K.L. et al. (2004) Women's reasons for not participating in follow up visits before starting short course antiretroviral prophylaxis for prevention of mother to child transmission of HIV: qualitative interview study. *British Medical Journal* 329 (7465), 543.

MY HUSBAND DOESN'T KNOW:

INVOLVING MALE PARTNERS IN MICROBICIDE RESEARCH

FACILITATOR'S NOTES

This case study is about a woman who decides to take part in a microbicide study without first telling her husband. It invites students to think beyond research participants as individual actors, and to reflect on how taking part in research may affect family relationships, and be affected by them. In the discussion you may wish to guide the group to think about decision-making practices in general in your community. Who has the power to make decisions in families? How is this different from the assumptions about individual decision-making made in the standard informed consent process? When designing research studies, are there ways to reconcile different ideas about decision-making and individual autonomy? For example, one possible solution might be to provide detailed information about the research to the community as a whole, so that men have some general facts even if their partners decide not to disclose their personal involvement.

The further reading provided for this case study gives a detailed exploration of partner dynamics in relation to microbicide use in Africa. It is worth reading alongside the case study for deeper reflection on how we conceptualize safe sex methods, and research into these.

LEARNING OBJECTIVE

To understand that although informed consent is often individual, participants have relationships (such as marriage) which may be affected by involvement in research

KEYWORDS

Informed consent

Partner involvement

Gender

MY HUSBAND DOESN'T KNOW:

INVOLVING MALE PARTNERS IN MICROBICDE RESEARCH

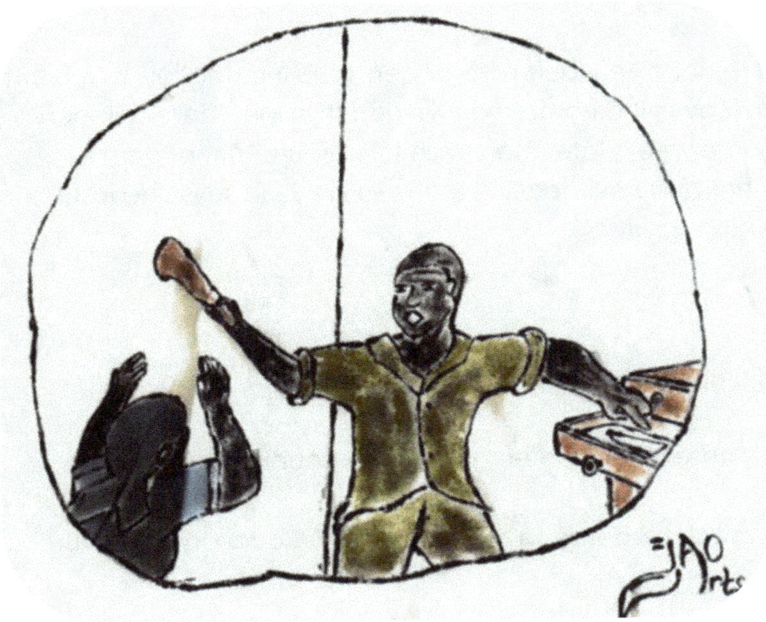

'WHERE DID YOU GET THIS THING?!' MARYBELLE'S HUSBAND FINDS HER MICROBICIDE GEL

THE STORY

Marybelle is taking part in a trial of a microbicide gel to see if it will protect women from HIV infection. She learns about the study when researchers come to the hotel where she is a cook. They tell her about the study and ask if she wants to participate. Marybelle is told that some women will receive the active gel and some will receive the placebo, but they won't be told which one they had. Marybelle decides to take part in the study because 'you can never tell what your husband may be doing'. She thinks the gel might offer her some protection from HIV infection, as her husband does not want to use condoms.

Following consultation with women participants in a pilot study, the trial staff decide not to involve women's partners in the trial in any way, except to offer to provide a referral to an STD clinic if desired. Women are encouraged to inform their partners about their participation in the trial, and about the gel, but receive no suggestions about how to do this.

At the time, Marybelle decides not to tell her husband about the gel at first. She isn't sure what his reaction would be, and feels it might bring some problems in her marriage, so she hides the gel. But one day, her husband finds it. He sees it has something to do with sex, and accuses her of having a boyfriend; he becomes angry and violent. Marybelle tries to explain that she is taking part in a research study, but has difficulty explaining the details.

On her next clinic visit she confides in her 'follow-up' worker, Maureen, who offers to talk to Marybelle's husband. Marybelle is doubtful that her husband will come to the clinic himself, so Maureen visits their home to talk to him.

During the visit, Marybelle's husband remains very quiet. He accepts the information sheet, but does not ask any questions. Maureen leaves the home a bit worried that Marybelle will soon withdraw from the study. However, some weeks later Marybelle tells Maureen that her husband has read the information sheet and now 'really likes the study'. She says: 'He just needed to take his time, and understand slowly.'

QUESTIONS

- Why do you think Marybelle did not tell her husband at first?
- Who are the participants in this case? The women alone? The couples? Why?
- What do you think about Maureen's response to the challenge? Could anything else have been done?
- Why did the research programme not seek husbands' consent? What disadvantages could there be to asking husbands for consent?
- What impact do you think husbands' consent (or lack of consent) might have on the research findings?
- How far do you think study staff are responsible for ensuring that male partners are provided with clear information about the gel?
- How much and in what way should information be provided to men, to ensure women's autonomy and prevent negative consequences? Do you think women and men need to be informed, or give consent, in the same ways? Can you think of any creative solutions?
- Can you think of other types of project where researchers' relationships may be affected by, or may affect, the study?

REFLECTION ON YOUR OWN EXPERIENCES

Can you think of similar situations from your experience? How did you ensure participants were at minimal risk of harm? Looking back now, what could you have done differently?

FURTHER READING

Montgomery, C.M. et al. (2008) The role of partnership dynamics in determining the acceptability of condoms and microbicides. *AIDS Care* 20(6), 733–740.

OF COURSE WE SPEAK ENGLISH:

COMMUNITY ENGAGEMENT AND DISSEMINATING INFORMATION

FACILITATOR'S NOTES

Community Advisory Boards (CABs) made up of local 'opinion leaders' are often a key part of community engagement activities. However, it is important to reflect carefully on the way researchers and people in the community communicate and relate to one another. In this story, CAB members do not readily comprehend the study information, yet the researchers are unaware of this. On a superficial level this is about the language used, but underlying this is a deeper issue of power. In the discussion you may wish to consider how the CAB members see the researchers, and what this might mean for transparency when the two groups interact.

LEARNING OBJECTIVE

To appreciate the challenges involved in communicating with people of different cultural, linguistic, educational, and socio-economic backgrounds, and to consider how these could be addressed in your context

KEYWORDS

Community engagement

Dissemination

Translation

OF COURSE WE SPEAK ENGLISH:
COMMUNITY ENGAGEMENT AND DISSEMINATING INFORMATION

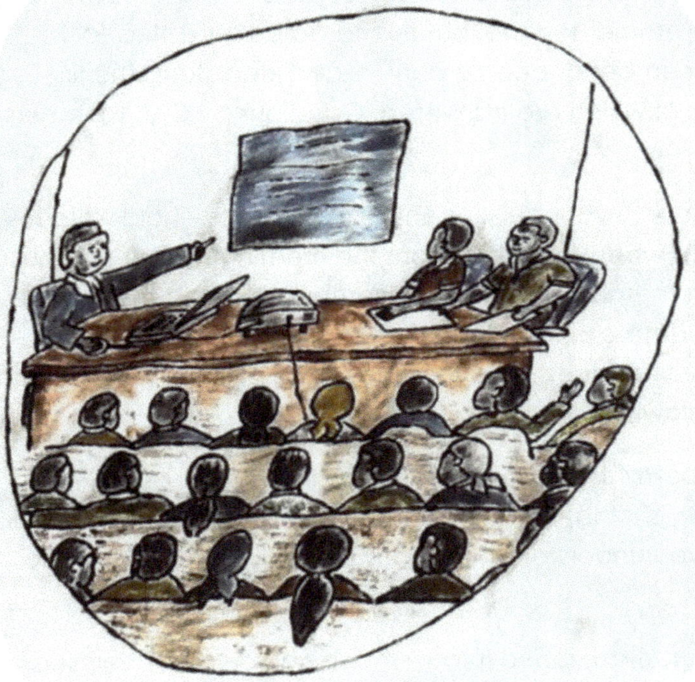

'UM... I HAVE A QUESTION: WHAT ON EARTH ARE YOU TALKING ABOUT?'

THE STORY

A Community Advisory Board (CAB) made up of local 'opinion leaders' is attached to an international research station. The CAB members are chosen on the basis of their standing in different groups in the local community: women, teachers, the local administration, religious leaders, people living with HIV/AIDS, etc. The researchers at the station believe these are people who are respected by others in these groups, and are able to explain the research to them as well as raise any concerns or questions from these communities. A condition of joining the CAB is a 'basic' ability to read, write and speak in English.

The research station operates in a part of Africa where there are several languages used: English, a national language, and a tribal 'mother-tongue'. With so much variation, the situation is made more complicated because people who appear to be speaking the same language might have different levels of skill and different styles. A highly educated scientist living in town but able to speak mother-tongue, for example, may not speak what local people call the 'deep' mother-tongue used by villagers. Equally, the English used by villagers might not be the same as the formal English used in scientific work.

At one particular CAB meeting, several research staff present their new studies to the CAB members. They all use different language combinations, but their PowerPoint slides are written in English. One of the speakers tries to use mother-tongue, but this has to be repeated (or re-translated) by another, more local, staff member as people can't really understand the first time. The other speakers use English, parts of which are translated. Questions by CAB members are usually asked in English.

The next day, a visiting social scientist – a much younger student from overseas – holds a focus group with the CAB members, asking them what they learnt from the meeting. Out of the four projects discussed, the focus group only remember one. They remember all about the disease, which captured their interest, but not the details of the study. They say that there were too many studies discussed, they weren't given handouts, and that they were people 'long out of school', so they 'need to be taken more slowly'.

The English-speaking social scientist asks them if they found understanding the English difficult. They were indignant! 'No, we all speak English, that's why we were chosen!' 'True,' she says, 'but there are lots of kinds of English. Did you understand me today, when I welcomed you to this discussion?'

'Well, no,' they reply. 'But Amy [the translator] explained it too.' The social scientist is horrified. 'But you didn't tell me! I talked for a long time, and you were all nodding, looking like you were understanding me.' 'Well, yes,' they say. 'But you were trying hard. And anyway – we speak English too.'

A discussion in English then starts up among the CAB members. The CAB Chairman rebukes some members for just 'pretending' to be 'learned', and suggests that these people step down in response to the social scientist's comments. 'No,' the social scientist says, 'I was telling you I think you should step *up*, and feel free to say if you don't understand.'

QUESTIONS

- How would you describe what happened here? What are the key ethical issues?
- Why do you think knowledge of English was a requirement for the CAB? Should it be?
- Was language the only factor in the CAB members' not remembering the study facts? What other things might have played a role?

- Why do you think the CAB members were reluctant to say during the meeting itself that they were finding it difficult to understand?
- How about the focus group – could there be different reasons for why they didn't say they weren't understanding the social scientist at the start?
- What do you think about the CAB chair's response to the problem? What could this tell the researchers about the community?
- Does the limited comprehension of the CAB members matter? What might it mean for the research, both ethically, and in terms of scientific accuracy?
- Moving forward, how could communication between the CAB and the researchers be improved?

REFLECTION ON YOUR OWN EXPERIENCES

- Can you think of any similar situations from your experience? How did you deal with them? Looking back now, what could you have done differently?
- This case shows that translation can be more complicated than just using a dictionary. Accent, local styles, idioms, turns of phrase and so on can also be crucial. What does this mean for the way we translate study documents like consent forms, brochures, etc.?

SATANISTS OR SCIENTISTS?: DEALING WITH NEGATIVE ASSOCIATIONS

FACILITATOR'S NOTES

The purpose of this case study is to invite reflection on ethical approaches for individuals and for research organizations when addressing community concerns. The story relates what happens when a peer recruiter comes under fire through a new rumour about the research, and begins to have doubts herself. This case study points to the challenges faced by community engagement personnel, especially those from the local area, and highlights the fact that many people juggle several co-existing interpretations of what research is about, irrespective of their level of education.

Rather than being dismissed for their factual inaccuracy, rumours can be understood as expressions of genuine concern about the means and purposes of foreign-funded medical research. Far from being 'backward', these can reflect very real historical 'truths' about encounters between researchers and communities in a world of unequal relations.

LEARNING OBJECTIVE

To appreciate the importance of taking rumours seriously as expressions of genuine concern about the purpose of medical research, and a starting-point for debate – rather than dismissing them as naïve misunderstandings which obscure scientific 'truth'

KEYWORDS

Community engagement

Rumour

Blood

Peer educators

Money

SATANISTS OR SCIENTISTS?:
DEALING WITH NEGATIVE ASSOCIATIONS

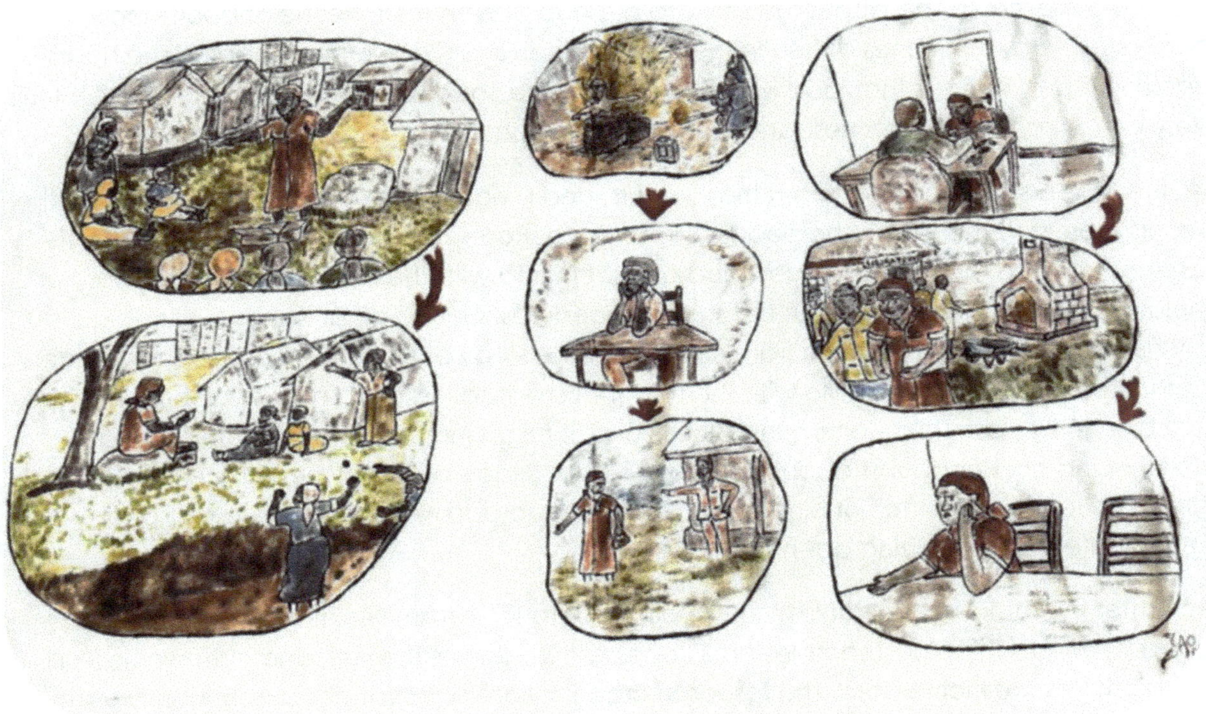

A WEEK IN THE LIFE OF ROSE: THE CHALLENGES OF BEING A PEER EDUCATOR

THE STORY

Rose has worked as a VCT (Voluntary HIV Counselling and Testing) counsellor for an NGO for some years when she hears about a new foreign-funded, one-year research project. The project will be a preparation study for a clinical trial of a new product, which aims to protect women against HIV infection. Rose joins the preparation study as one of the first participants. Because she speaks so freely about HIV to the other women in the waiting room, the staff invite her to become a peer educator on the project, and she accepts.

Rose considers herself lucky and takes her new job very seriously. She speaks about HIV and the project both in the research clinic and in her neighbourhood, recruiting many women for the study. The job does not come without its problems. People say that she must have HIV – otherwise, why does she like to speak about it so much? She's used to such rumours from her previous job, and she knows how and when to address them.

But Rose is less prepared for another rumour that begins to circulate after a while, suggesting that the researchers are associated with Satanists, and that they take blood from study participants to sell it abroad in order to prosper. Why, otherwise, would they need so much blood from participants, when an HIV test can be done with only one drop of blood? And why would people receive money just for coming to a clinic? Around this time, although not related directly to the project, an old woman is burnt alive in the street, accused of Satanism. When Rose is giving a talk about the study to a group of women in her neighbourhood, people start throwing stones at her. In the market when she is doing her shopping she hears people whisper, 'There's that lady who works with those Satanists. Her money is tainted.' All this is very unsettling, and Rose's husband wants her to quit her job.

The newspapers also find out about the rumours, and a national columnist comments that the rumours merely demonstrate the people's ignorance. Rose considers herself better educated than most, and so far, she has understood and identified with the information that her employers have offered her about the study procedures. On the other hand, she feels quite dizzy herself when blood is drawn from her arm for the study every three months. She wonders whether this has something to do with the fact that she had lost quite a lot of blood when she gave birth to her last child – or, on the other hand, it might indicate that something bad is indeed going on. Her doubts about the research are exacerbated by her memories of an older rumour about a batch of birth control pills from abroad, which had allegedly been contaminated by a sterilizing agent.

To counter the rumours of Satanism, the research organization invites all staff to visit the laboratory where the blood samples are processed. Rose joins the visit, and is shown how all blood samples are incinerated. The research organization also arranges a community meeting where study participants explain to their relatives and neighbours what the research project is about.

The rumours do lessen after this, but Rose is still asked occasionally why she works with the Satanists. When the preparation study is completed and the 'real' trial is about to begin, Rose is unsure about whether or not to join it.

QUESTIONS

- Do you think Rose discussed her concerns with her employers? If not, why not? How could her employers support her better?
- What can rumours tell us about relations between researchers and community? In this case, what real concerns are being expressed? What historical truths are being reflected?
- How can research organizations address the concerns that rumours raise?

REFLECTION ON YOUR OWN EXPERIENCES

- Have you come across rumours associated with medical research?
- How did these rumours influence your work?
- How were they addressed by your organization?
- Can you think of other ways to address the concerns which the rumours express?

ACTIVITY

Divide into groups of four to six and discuss the 'reflection' questions. Try to formulate guidelines on how a research organization could handle concerns and rumours about research.

FURTHER READING

Fairhead, J., Leach, M., and Small, M. (2006) Where techno-science meets poverty: medical research and the economy of blood in The Gambia, West Africa. *Social Science and Medicine*, 63(4), 1109–1120.

Feldman-Savelsberg, P., Ndonko, F.T., and Schmidt-Ehry, B. (2000) Sterilizing vaccines or the politics of the womb: retrospective study of a rumor in Cameroon. *Medical Anthropology Quarterly* 14, 159–179.

Geissler, P.W. (2005) 'Kachinja are coming!': encounters around medical research work in a Kenyan village. *Africa: Journal of the International African Institute* 75, 173–202.

Geissler, P.W. and Pool, R. (2006) Editorial: Popular concerns about medical research projects in sub-Saharan Africa – a critical voice in debates about medical research ethics. *Tropical Medicine & International Health* 11(7), 975–982. Available at: http://onlinelibrary.wiley.com/doi/10.1111/j.1365-3156.2006.01682.x/pdf (accessed 25 October 2015).

Kingori, P. et al. (2010) 'Rumours' and clinical trials: a retrospective examination of a paediatric malnutrition study in Zambia, southern Africa. *BMC Public Health* 10(1), 556.

THE SHEEP STUDY:
OLD MEMORIES OF FOOD, BLOOD AND DEATH

FACILITATOR'S NOTES

This story is designed to encourage you to think about how communities remember research. In some communities, research has been conducted for many years, sometimes by several different organizations. What effect does this have on how such communities perceive studies? Sometimes researchers complain that participants suffer from being 'over researched' or from 'research fatigue'. This story asks your students to think more widely about how memories of past research might inform perceptions of current or future research. It also asks readers to consider what messages former research participants are left with. Dissemination of research findings is seen as a key aspect of good research, but what will participants remember several years down the line?

In exploring this, the story also raises an important point about rumours around medical research. Other case studies in this collection stress that rumours should be understood more as a social commentary on living conditions, rather than as 'misinformation'. Here, we add an additional historical dimension. Rumours about current medical research may speak to collective memories of both past research, and rumours about it.

LEARNING OBJECTIVE

To raise awareness of the impact of community memories of previous research on the success of future research

KEYWORDS

Inducements
Rumour
Adverse events
Blood
Long-term engagement
Memories of past research

THE SHEEP STUDY:
OLD MEMORIES OF FOOD, BLOOD AND DEATH

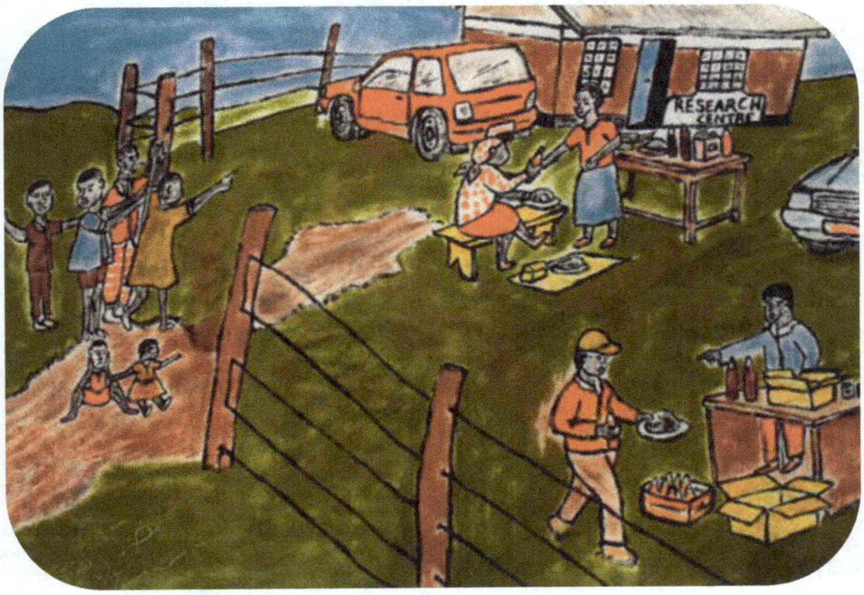

THE CHILDREN WERE CURIOUS – WHAT KIND OF STRANGE PARTY WAS THIS?

THE STORY

In this rural part of a Central African country, transnational medical research has been conducted by a range of agencies for many years. One of the first studies in the region is collectively remembered as 'the Sheep Study'. The actual purpose and routines of the research are long forgotten. What people do remember – or have heard about from their parents and grandparents – is that researchers came and cooked a feast for the research participants every single day. Villagers who were young children at the time remember standing at the research compound's fence, and watching cooks prepare luxury foods like chapati, liver and, most importantly, roasted lamb. These were rare foods, normally reserved for funerals or Christmas. One young woman remembers her mother keeping her away from the compound for fear that she would be kidnapped by the researchers. Those who participated in the research remember visiting the compound every day to 'take their drugs', which they washed down with soda and the feast.

Why did the researchers prepare this feast for the participants? The collective memory is that the drugs were very 'harsh'. They couldn't be taken on an empty stomach, and at that time of national famine, stomachs were *very* empty. What happened to that research? The villagers recall it ended somewhat prematurely. People have heard that some participants died some years after the study, because the drugs were 'too strong'. What happened to the researchers? They left. Very few people can remember the name of the research organization. Just that some of the people in charge were white.

One of the former local research assistants has a better memory. He recalls that the British Principal Investigator had insisted on providing the good food. Some of the staff, he says, had told him that that's what people would expect to eat. The research assistant also remembers that, at the time, he thought providing such festive food might make people suspicious. 'They'll wonder what they have to exchange for such a good meal!' But he didn't say anything to the Principal Investigator.

After the Sheep Study finished, the researchers left the area and a new research organization came in. Although most people today know the name of the newer organization, they aren't clear that they weren't also responsible for the Sheep Study. Occasionally, when rumours surface around new research projects, people remember and talk about the people who supposedly died after taking part in the Sheep Study.

QUESTIONS

- What does this case study tell us about the ways that participants might remember research studies?
- Why do you think the villagers remember the food more than the research itself?
- Do you think the memories of the Sheep Study matter, both practically (for the new project) and ethically?
- What could the new research organization do to distance itself from the Sheep Study?

REFLECTIONS ON YOUR OWN EXPERIENCES

- What procedures are in place for governing collaboration between research organizations in your area?
- Do organizations share their experiences with each other? Are there systems in place to streamline the way researchers communicate about what they are doing with the community? What is the role of research, and the role of the government, in promoting this?
- Have you worked on a research project where former participants remember the 'wrong thing' about the study? What kind of things do they tend to remember? What do they forget? What dissemination have you done or could you do to change this?

FURTHER READING

Fairhead, J., Leach, M., and Small, M. (2006) Where techno-science meets poverty: medical research and the economy of blood in The Gambia, West Africa. *Social Science and Medicine*, 63(4), 1109–1120.

Geissler, P.W. (2005) 'Kachinja are coming!': encounters around medical research work in a Kenyan village. *Africa: Journal of the International African Institute* 75, 173–202.

Geissler, P.W. and Pool, R. (2006) Editorial: Popular concerns about medical research projects in sub-Saharan Africa – a critical voice in debates about medical research ethics. *Tropical Medicine & International Health* 11(7), 975–982. Available at: http://onlinelibrary.wiley.com/doi/10.1111/j.1365-3156.2006.01682.x/pdf (accessed 25 October 2015.)

Kingori, P. et al. (2010) 'Rumours' and clinical trials: a retrospective examination of a paediatric malnutrition study in Zambia, southern Africa. *BMC Public Health* 10(1), 556.

WILL THEY LEAVE US WHERE WE ARE?: EXPECTATIONS OF MEDICAL RESEARCH INTERVENTIONS

FACILITATOR'S NOTES

This story highlights the fact that medical research projects often share similarities with projects which try to create more immediate change in local communities. For example, when compared with NGOs and 'development' bodies which have a primary goal of improving current conditions, they may have a similar physical presence, comparable organizational structures and practices, and project activities which seem the same to local people. Such similarities may create expectations about the goals of the work, and hopes for immediate changes.

The purpose of this story is not to discuss how research organizations and their staff should correct this 'misunderstanding'. Rather, the case aims to suggest that it might be more ethical for research organizations to adopt more 'developmental' goals, aiming to create both immediate and lasting change, as resource-rich and often long-term collaborators within both a local community and a national health system.

LEARNING OBJECTIVE

To consider similarities between medical research and other kinds of community interventions, the expectations that these similarities may create, and the possible ways that research organizations could address these issues

KEYWORDS

Long-term engagement
Community engagement
Memories of past research

WILL THEY LEAVE US WHERE WE ARE?:

EXPECTATIONS OF MEDICAL RESEARCH INTERVENTIONS

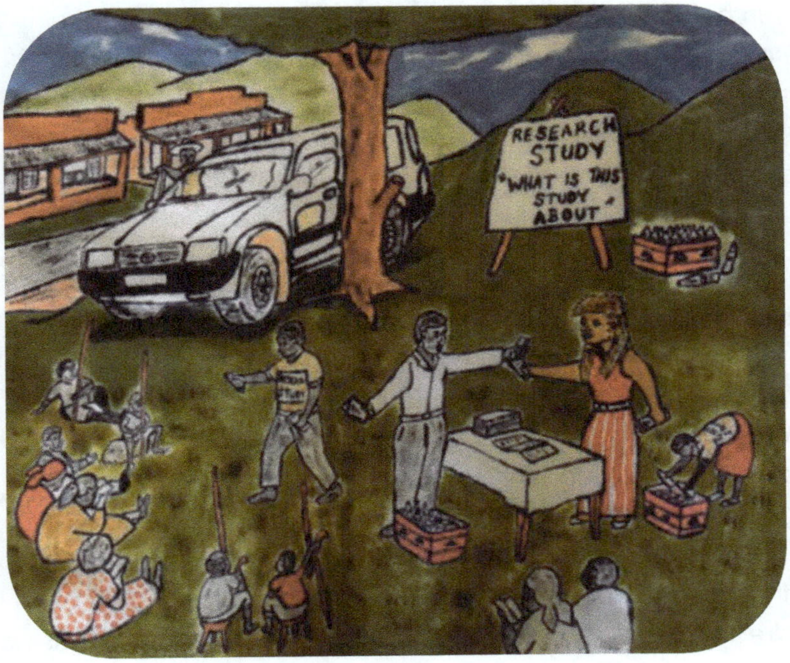

'YES, WHAT REALLY IS THIS ALL ABOUT?' WONDERED LINDA

THE STORY

Linda has no formal job, but she and her husband have built some rooms to rent in the urban shanty town where they live. With her children grown up, and more time on her hands, she has become an experienced volunteer in a public health clinic, where she is elected a member of the Neighbourhood Health Committee. The sister-in-charge at the clinic often sends her to workshops and seminars on various health programmes because Linda is so good at communicating what she has learnt to her fellow volunteers. She is trained as a child health promoter, and helps distribute food donated by various international agencies among families with malnourished children. She is active in her church choir, which often receives visitors from abroad, and she also works in one of the local community schools. This school is run by a local NGO which has strong connections to an international NGO with offices in the city. She likes the way that those involved with the school seem to gain training and opportunities.

Linda is hardworking and very well connected. Because of these connections she is also very well informed about what is going on in the community – including what programmes are coming to the area. She does her best to share her knowledge and connections with people in her neighbourhood. To use a common local expression, she 'has a heart for the community'.

Because of her position, she is among the first to learn of a new project that is to start at the clinic. It is an HIV research project, run by an NGO working with the government to improve public health. Linda is ready at the clinic on the first day that local participant recruiters are being hired, and she is selected and joins the training. She learns about the purpose and the time-frame of the project, and the various activities that will take place. She then begins her job recruiting and retaining study participants, and entering various kinds of data into the project computers. She enjoys the project meetings, where she learns a great deal and meets many influential people.

Linda can't help noticing the different ways in which the research organization interacts with people's lives and job prospects. She receives a salary for her work as long as the project lasts. It's a relatively high and much more stable income than she usually gets. Community representatives on the liaison board established by the organization are not paid, but receive allowances for meetings, various local training opportunities, and access to computer and Internet facilities in the meeting room. As for medical personnel, a young doctor Linda knows from the clinic is also hired to work for the research organization, and receives a lot of training abroad, ending up with a degree from a foreign university. At the same time, nurses working in local public clinics are sometimes hired by the researchers, but when the project finally ends after several years, they find it difficult to get a position in their old organizations.

When the project ends, Linda finds things are much the same as when it started. People are still getting sick with HIV and dying. All her years of effort have provided some extra income, but created little change in the community, and given her nothing to help her move into another similar job. Looking back, Linda feels less positive about overseas research projects than before. Talking about projects with her many contacts, she starts to express the opinion that the foreign researchers 'come and take our information and then leave. They leave us where we are, without empowering us. If we volunteer for them we don't get trained so that we can get a job afterwards.'

QUESTIONS

- What are some of the similarities between medical research organizations and other projects which might operate in local communities? What are the differences? Consider the organizations' structure, physical presence, employment and recruitment strategies, and goals.

- What do you think about the way the research organization treats the different people who get involved? Do you think this might create problems? If so, for whom?

- Why do you think it is difficult for local health workers to move between the public health system and the international research project?

- What do you think about Linda's expectations of the project? Do you think she should be satisfied with her experience? Or should the research organization do more to address immediate problems in the area?

- Should the research organization start to pay all its participants? What might this mean in terms of practicalities on the ground, the quality of data, and research ethics?

- Are there other ways the research organization could try to alleviate poverty in the area, in order to limit some of these problems? How far do you think a research organization should go in assisting the wider community?

- Who do you think should be involved in deciding on the objectives of overseas projects in local areas?

REFLECTION ON YOUR OWN EXPERIENCE

- Have you come across expectations about medical research projects, which your organization had not planned for?

- How did your organization respond? Could things have been done differently?

SEEING IS BELIEVING:
TRIAL REGULATIONS VS. COMMUNITY ENGAGEMENT IN AN EBOLA VACCINE TRIAL

FACILITATOR'S NOTES

The story, set in the context of an Ebola outbreak, focuses on the difficulty of balancing internationally agreed protocols with demands in the field and the nature of social relationships between local staff and community members. Ethical guidelines can often feel detached from the realities of everyday interactions and can put staff working on clinical trials in difficult positions when the demands of the trial run counter to those of social relations on the ground. There are three key issues to be explored in this case study.

The first has to do with the fact that employees in an Ebola vaccine trial are not allowed to take the trial vaccine. The study coordinator calls this the 'conflict of interest rule.' The idea behind this is that employees may feel pressured to take the vaccine that their employer is trialing, and this would put in question the voluntary nature of their participation. In the context of an outbreak, this restriction for local staff inevitably raises concerns that do not arise when clinical trials are being done outside of epidemic settings. The case study thus requires the reader to think about how standardised ethical protocols may present different questions depending on the context in which they are taking place.

Secondly, the market trader's insistence that 'seeing is believing', brings up the issue of trust and social relations. The fact that two trial staff, John and Jane, are from the community where the trial is taking place and that, Hawa the market trader, is Jane's mother in law should lead us to reflect on the complexity of social relationships and the challenges faced by local staff when attempting to navigate the difficult terrains of community engagement in vaccine trials.

LEARNING OBJECTIVE

To explore the challenges of balancing the demands of internationally agreed protocols with demands in the field during an epidemic

KEYWORDS

Rumour
Study rules
Recruitment
Community-based fieldworkers
Community engagement
Outbreak

Community members' concerns with the fact that local trial staff cannot take the vaccine should also prompt the reader to think through motives for participating in vaccine trials and the prominent role played by social relations and trust in community members employed by the study - especially under conditions of an outbreak or emergency.

Finally, the emergence of a rumour surrounding the potentially sinister motives of the vaccine trials depicts how anxieties surrounding vaccine trials - amplified by an epidemic – can be articulated through hearsay and how they can be understood as products of fears and mistrust. Furthermore, Jane's difficult personal experiences and her suggestion that perhaps she ought to lie about her ability to take the vaccine also suggest the very real worries that rumours create amongst trial staff both in terms of their potential impact on the running of the trial itself but also, and more importantly, in terms of the damage that they may cause to social relationships that will outlive the presence of the trial in the community.

SEEING IS BELIEVING:
TRIAL REGULATIONS VS. COMMUNITY ENGAGEMENT IN AN EBOLA VACCINE TRIAL

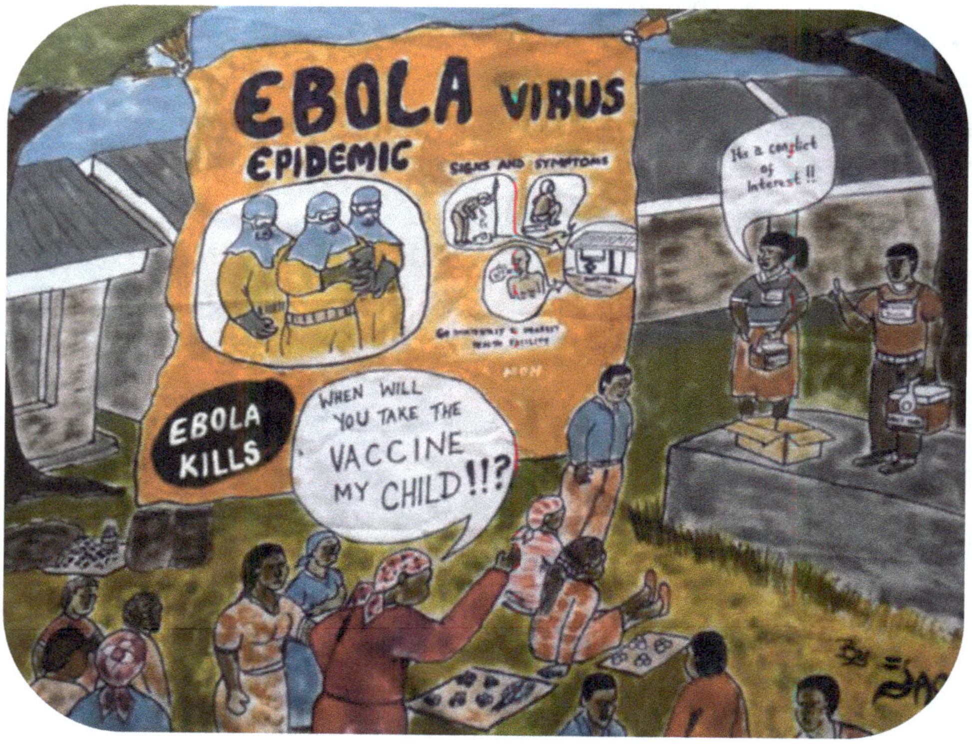
EBOLA VIRUS
EPIDEMIC
SIGNS AND SYMPTOMS
It's a conflict of interest!!
EBOLA KILLS
WHEN WILL YOU TAKE THE VACCINE MY CHILD!!?

'WHEN WILL *YOU* TAKE THE VACINE MY CHILD?!'

THE STORY

John and Jane are community liaison officers in an Ebola vaccine trial taking place in the middle of an Ebola epidemic. Because they are employed by the trial, John and Jane are told by their managers that they cannot receive the vaccine candidate, as it would constitute a conflict of interest'. They are not entirely sure what this means. Despite their concerns about contracting the disease and their disappointment about not being able to receive the vaccine, John and Jane decide that they really want to be involved in the fight against the virus in their own community, and continue to work for the project.

As the trial gets underway, John and Jane are asked to organize community meetings to introduce the vaccine and to explain the modalities of the trial, including the fact that participation is entirely voluntary. Their first meeting is with a group of market traders and is held in the hall of the town's market. After having given a short presentation about the trial, John and Jane open up the floor for questions. The first to ask a question is Hawa, the leader of the market traders – and Jane's mother in law. Hawa asks when the traders can expect to see Jane, John and all of their colleagues receiving the Ebola vaccine. "Seeing is believing", she adds, and says that once they have seen them take the vaccine publicly, people in the town will feel more confident in taking part in the trial. Jane and John look towards their supervisor, who nods to suggest they must tell the audience about the conflict of interest rule that prevents them from taking the vaccine. Once they have finished explaining, Hawa asks: "But you are our children, how do you expect us to take this if you won't?"

A few days after the meeting, rumours begin spreading that the trial vaccine is a slow poison, which will infect those who take it with Ebola to cause another epidemic in a few years' time. This, the rumour goes, is the reason why trial staff will not take the vaccine publicly. The study coordinator calls John and Jane to a meeting to discuss ways of addressing these concerns. At the meeting, Jane tells the coordinator about the market trader meeting, and that her mother in law has stopped talking to her and that people in her compound no longer trust her. She asks if they can tell the community that trial staff will in fact be allowed to take the vaccine in the near future.

QUESTIONS

- What are the ethical issues at stake?
- What do you think is the 'conflict of interest' alluded to that excludes staff from receiving the trial vaccine?
- What do you think about the decision of excluding staff from the trial during an epidemic? Do you agree or disagree? Why?
- Why do you think it was so important to Hawa that Jane and John take the vaccine in front of community members? Do you think it is fair of Hawa to expect Jane and John to take the vaccine?
- How can we explain the rumours emerging in town after the meeting with the market traders?
- What do you make of Jane's suggestion that she tells the community staff will take the vaccine later? Why do you think it is important to her that the community thinks she will be taking the vaccine at a later stage?
- What are the possible responses the study coordinator could give to Jane's idea?

REFLECTIONS ON YOUR OWN EXPERIENCE

- Have you experienced anything similar? How have you dealt with the possibility of losing community members' trust?
- Can you think of any other examples where the trial's regulations come into conflict with local staff's commitments to their communities?
- What are the key ethical differences between a trial under outbreak conditions and a routine trial on prevention or treatment of endemic disease?

ACTIVITY

Divide into groups of 4 and devise a community liaison strategy for countering rumours that the vaccine is slow poison and a communication strategy around why trial staff are not allowed to take the vaccine.

FURTHER READING

Marsh, V., Kamuya, D., Mlamba, A., Williams, S., Molyneux, S. (2010) Experiences with community engagement and informed consent in a genetic cohort study of severe childhood diseases in Kenya. *BMC Medical Ethics*, 11-13.

Global Campaign for Microbicides (2004) *Mobilization for Community Involvement in Microbicides Trials: A Report from a Dialogue in Southern Africa*. Washington DC, USA. Accessed 27th June 2016: http://www.global-campaign.org/clientfiles/SA-community-involvement.pdf

Larson, H., Cooper, L., Eskola, J., Katz, S., Ratzan, S. (2011) Addressing the Vaccine Confidence Gap. *The Lancet* 378:9790, 526–535.

Hantel, A., Olopade, CO. (2015) Drug and Vaccine Access in the Ebola Epidemic: Advising Caution in Compassionate Use. *Ann Intern Med* 162, 141-142.

ANTHROPOLOGY AND EBOLA WEB RESOURCES

The Ebola Response Anthropology Platform: http://www.ebola-anthropology.net/ . Accessed 27th June 2016.

Series of anthropological blogs on Ebola: http://somatosphere.net/series/ebola-fieldnotes . Accessed 27th June 2016.

Anthropology and Ebola Communication page on the Ebola Communication Network website: http://ebolacommunicationnetwork.org/anthropology-and-ebola-communication/ Accessed 27th June 2016.

INSTITUTIONAL RELATIONSHIPS

TRAINING CASE STUDIES

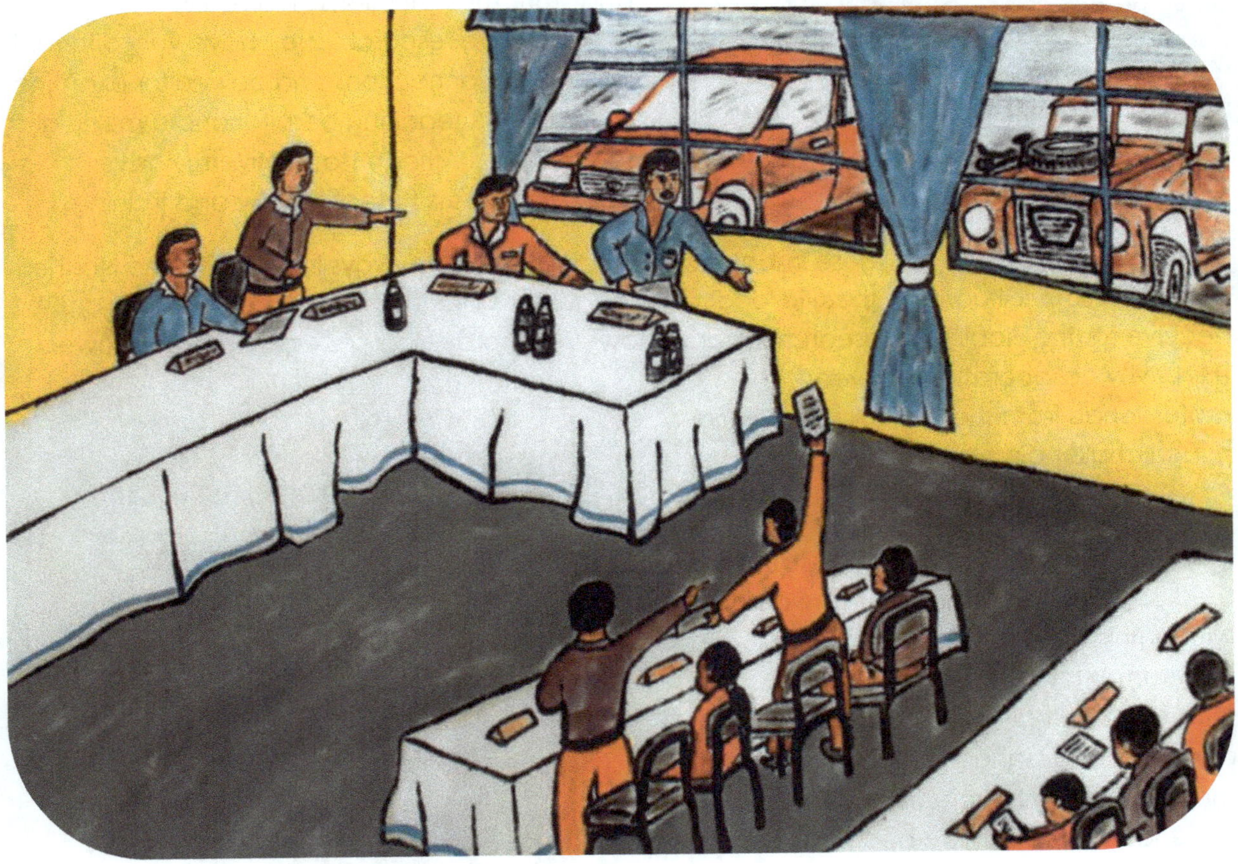

'DO TOO MANY COOKS SPOIL THE BROTH OR MAKE IT BETTER?' WONDERED THE CHAIR OF THE RESEARCH STAKEHOLDERS FORUM

INSTITUTIONAL RELATIONSHIPS

CASE STUDIES

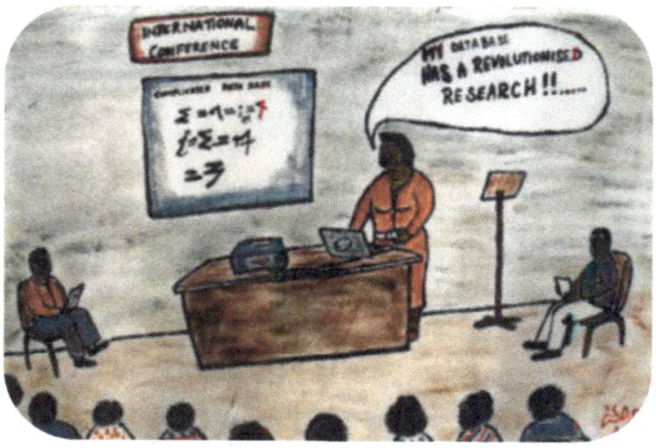

MY DATA OR ***OUR*** DATA?

Global health research relies on a series of collaborations: collaborations between countries, governments, institutions, funders and agencies – all with their own logics, agendas and staff. The institutions involved in collaborative research often have very different resources, connections and power; for example, a leading US teaching hospital and a medical faculty at an African state university have different access to technology and training. These imbalances are often but not always in favour of the Northern partner; in some situations, specific local knowledge or political and other connections can be decisive for the viability of research. Overall, however, more resources equal greater power. This is why collaboration between professionals from these different institutions is such challenging terrain.

In addition to scientific institutions and universities, transnational collaborative medical research often involves working with, within, or in consultation with government health services. In this context, differences in training, expectations, resources and standards of care between medical research projects and local healthcare facilities can be sources of tension in official relationships. Many of the case studies in this section are stories about this. How can and should research handle these healthcare-related differences? How can we both conduct good research, and contribute to good public health in these circumstances?

FURTHER READING

Lairumbi, G.M. et al. (2008) Promoting the social value of research in Kenya: examining the practical aspects of collaborative partnerships using an ethical frame. *Social Science and Medicine* 67(5), 734–47.

Moyi Okwaro, F. and Geissler, P. W. (2015). In/dependent Collaborations: Perceptions and Experiences of African Scientists in Transnational HIV Research. *Medical Anthropology Quarterly* 29, 492–511

Lachenal, G et al (2016) Neglected Actors in Neglected Tropical Diseases Research: Historical Perspectives on Health Workers and Contemporary Buruli Ulcer Research in Ayos, Cameroon. *PLoS Neglected Tropical Disease* 10(4): e0004488

TOO MANY PEOPLE HAVE TURNED UP!

ADDRESSING STAKEHOLDERS' CONCERNS

FACILITATOR'S NOTES

This case study is about relationships between collaborative research programmes on the one hand, and government officials and other local stakeholders on the other. In the story, researchers aim to respond constructively to complaints about their work, but their efforts do not seem to solve the immediate problem. How can research organizations develop constructive and mutually beneficial collaborations in this type of setting, without placing themselves under unreasonable obligation, or going beyond their remit and responsibility?

The story raises questions about divergent obligations and expectations, and also about power relations, including the sovereignty of both local officials and the researchers. Questions about power, transparency, communication, obligations, and expectations are at the heart of this story, and are likely to emerge in your discussion.

You could also consider the main criticisms raised by the senior government official in the story, and discuss them one by one. Your discussion should acknowledge that some of these comments include an implicit appeal for access to resources and 'fringe benefits', and consider how the research organization could respond.

LEARNING OBJECTIVE

To consider ways of developing constructive and mutually beneficial relationships with local collaborators, given differing priorities and the limits of a research organization's responsibility and resources

KEYWORDS

Community entry

Government

Corruption

TOO MANY PEOPLE HAVE TURNED UP!:

ADDRESSING STAKEHOLDERS' CONCERNS

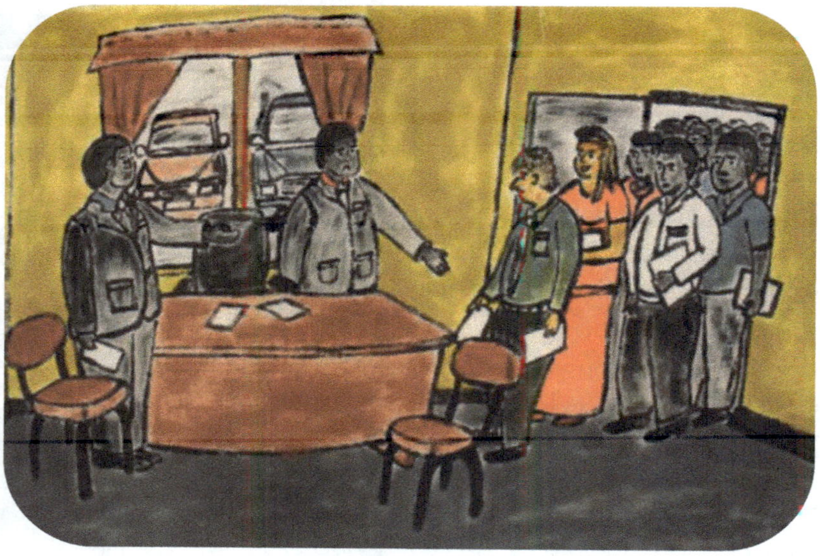

SUDDENLY THE ROOM FELT A LITTLE CROWDED!

THE STORY

Sarah is a community relations officer at a large international research centre which operates in a rural area of Malawi. The research at this field station includes demographic health surveillance, malaria research, and HIV treatment and prevention studies.

In the course of Sarah's work, she attends a 'health stakeholders' forum' every three months, where she is frequently attacked with numerous questions. These are mostly about the way the research collaboration operates, how it is financed, why it does not collaborate more with local universities and NGOs, and why senior staff haven't visited senior officials. At one meeting, the senior government officer who is acting as chair requests that the national and international directors of the research programme arrange to see him next week. By the time the meeting closes, it is late on Friday afternoon, and it takes Sarah another hour to return to the main research offices by Land Cruiser.

On Monday morning Sarah informs the national and international director about the complaints voiced at the meeting. A large group of senior international and national researchers and administrators are immediately dispatched to visit the senior government officer in two Land Cruisers. En route, Sarah tries to ring his office to inform him that they are coming, but the mobile network is down and she cannot get through. During the journey the team try to understand what has led to this situation. One African scientist comments, 'It is well within the senior government officer's jurisdiction to close the research programme down.'

It is about 10.30 when the team arrive at the governmental offices. The senior government officer is out at meetings, but due back shortly. His secretary tells the team to wait, and records everyone's name in the appointments book. Before long, the senior officer arrives, and after greeting everyone his first comment is: 'Too many people have turned up.' With difficulty, his secretary finds enough chairs to accommodate everyone in his office.

During the introductions the senior government officer stresses that he has been in post for several months, and this is the first time that he has received a formal visit from anybody from the research centre. He starts by summarising the complaints voiced at the meeting, specifically highlighting the need for researchers not to bypass senior council and governmental leaders. He also explains that stakeholders from NGOs and local universities feel excluded from contributing to health development in the areas where the research collaboration operates.

The team reply that, since a lot of their research is community-based, they have primarily focused on establishing several community advisory boards, and consulting with local government officers. 'This is good, but not good enough,' the senior government officer responds. He sums up by saying, 'If you work in isolation you will have people fighting against you. We need a new start. How should we proceed?'

QUESTIONS

- What were local stakeholders' concerns about the research programme?
- Why do you think the stakeholders raised these issues in the way they did?
- Do you think Sarah should attend the stakeholder forum meetings alone? What do you think this says about how seriously the research organization takes stakeholder engagement?
- Do you think the research organization should take the requests 'at face value', or do you think the comments may have contained underlying demands, which were not stated clearly? What do you think these might be?
- What do you think the senior government officer expected to see happen after the stakeholders' meeting, both immediately and in the longer term? Do you think things went as he expected?

- What do you think about the research organization's response to the stakeholders' complaints? Why were so many people from the research programme dispatched to see the senior government officer? Do you think this was a good idea?
- Why do you think the senior government officer might have been concerned about the number of people who turned up? What does this tell you about his intentions?
- What do you think about his comment about local healthcare provision in the area?
- What were a) the researchers and b) the senior government officer trying to get across in the meeting?
- How do you think the government official could 'close down' the programme if he decided to?
- How should the director of the research collaboration respond to this situation now?
- Do you think there is a need for 'personal relationships' even in community-led projects, and if so, how far do these extend?
- Do you think research organizations should try to work with in-country institutions such as NGOs and universities? Why?
- Do you think that local and national government officers should have a say over how research operates? If so, how do you think this should work? What kind of projects would this be more, and less, appropriate for?

ACTIVITY

Split into groups of four to six and try to develop a community engagement strategy, with a particular focus on how you will involve leaders from the local government administration. Think carefully about how to support collaboration, and how to negotiate explicit and implicit expectations.

FURTHER READING

Emanuel, E.J., Wendler, D., Killen, J., and Grady, C. (2004) What makes clinical research in developing countries ethical? The benchmarks of ethical research. *Journal of Infectious Disease* 189, 930–937.

Meslin, E.M. (2008) Achieving global justice in health through global research ethics: supplementing Macklin's 'top-down' approach with one from the 'ground up'. In: Green, R.M., Donovan, A., and Jauss, S.A. (eds.) *Global Bioethics: Issues of Conscience for the Twenty-First Century*. Clarendon Press, Oxford, UK.

DATA TROUBLES:
COLLABORATION AND THE FUTURE OF PARTNERSHIP

FACILITATOR'S NOTES

This case study is about the nature of partnership in research collaborations, with a focus on equality and involvement in decision-making, and access to and use of patients' health data. It raises questions about the ownership of patients' health records, their purpose (clinical and scientific), how this data should be used, and who stands to benefit from this resource.

The ethics of data sharing, and the development of policies and guidelines to support practice, are currently receiving much due attention from regulatory bodies, bioethics councils and medical institutes. You can access more information about this consensus work via the links provided under 'Further Reading'. Please note, however, that this is an evolving discussion, so you may want to look into the most up-to-date guidance from these bodies. The topics discussed in this consensus work are very relevant to this case study. They include rules of engagement, protecting patient confidentiality, and the need for frameworks that facilitate the responsible sharing of clinical and trial data in the interests of public health.

Deciding on rules of engagement or drawing up memoranda of understanding is a critical process in research collaboration, and one that may need to be revisited and renegotiated over time. In the story below, the research relationship started informally and was established in a spirit of networking. Both parties benefited from this relationship: the doctor's workplace was improved and could serve more patients, and the scientist accessed valuable data to further his research. Over time, however, the doctor begins to sense that his therapeutic expertise is being sidelined in favour of

LEARNING OBJECTIVE

To explore access to, use, and ownership of participants' health data in collaborative medical research, and through this to reflect on collaboration between unequal partners

KEYWORDS

Ownership

Data sharing

North-South relationships

capturing research-quality data. He also starts to question the equality of the collaboration, given that the scientist assumes primary ownership of the data and fails to actively involve him in the dissemination of findings and plans for new studies. The fact that communication between both parties is very limited contributes to the deterioration of the relationship. In your session you could ask participants to think about how this situation could have been prevented, or rectified.

DATA TROUBLES:

COLLABORATION AND THE FUTURE OF PARTNERSHIP

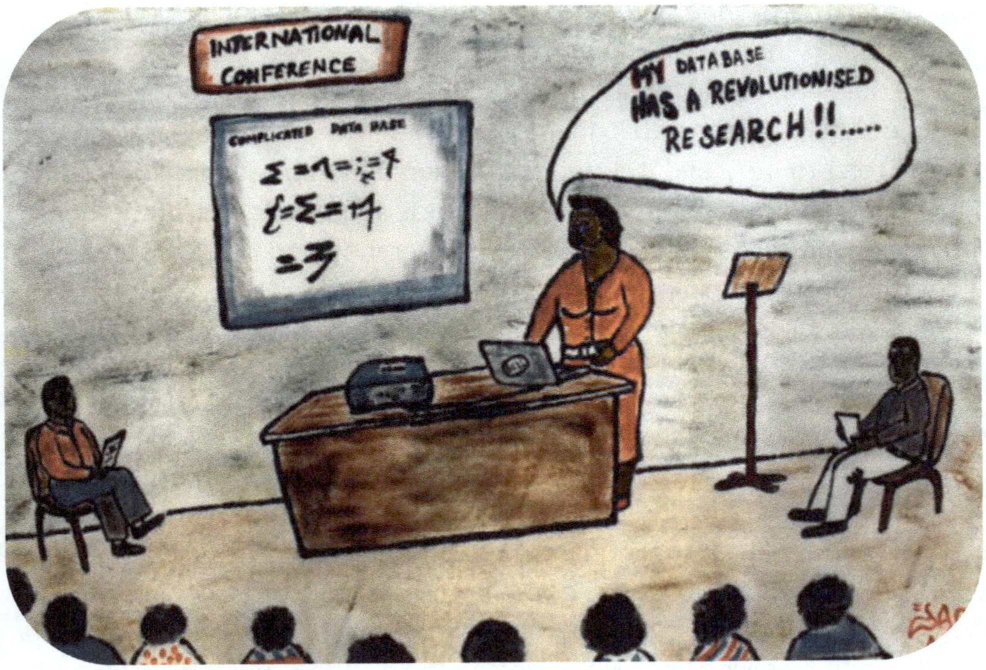
INTERNATIONAL CONFERENCE
COMPLICATED DATA BASE
MY DATABASE HAS A REVOLUTIONISED RESEARCH !!......

DR SEKIDDE WAITED PATIENTLY FOR THE ACKNOWLEDGEMENT THAT NEVER CAME

THE STORY

Musa Sekidde is a doctor in a local clinic. For about ten years, he has been keeping a register of his patients who are taking antiretroviral therapy. The ledger contains key information including each patient's identity, address, therapeutic regimen and disease progression.

About five years ago Dr Sekidde attended an HIV medicine training programme where he met Dr Martha Smith, a professor of medicine and epidemiology from a UK university. Dr Smith had been working in the capital but was looking for a clinic where she could conduct research among a rural population. She was very impressed with the detail and rigour of Dr Sekidde's bookkeeping and, after visiting Dr Sekidde's facility, Dr Smith proposed a research partnership. During the discussions, Dr Smith also promised to create and donate a computer database of patient records. Dr Sekidde accepted her proposal.

Initially, the collaboration worked well. Dr Smith's study was well-funded and Dr Sekidde's clinic was transformed from a basic facility to one that could accommodate several thousands of patients comfortably. However, despite these positive changes, a few things began to bother Dr Sekidde. For one thing, his clinical expertise was constantly being sidelined. Dr Smith was only interested in data that could be gathered through advanced diagnostic technologies (which she had also donated to the clinic), and she showed no interest in her colleague's clinical observations. In addition, while the computer-generated clinical forms looked 'smarter' then the exercise books that Dr Sekidde had used previously, they took considerable time to fill out, and missed out important information about the physical status of patients – details which were being carefully elaborated in the hand-written records. More troubling was that Dr Smith continued to refer to the patient database as 'hers' when presenting findings at a number of international conferences. While she always included Dr Sekidde as co-author, more often than not Dr Smith only shared the slides with him after they had been presented. Dr Smith had also mentioned to Dr Sekidde in passing that she was planning to apply for further funding to conduct studies with Dr Sekidde's patients, but a full proposal had not been formally discussed.

Things come to a head when a Norwegian research team approaches Dr Sekidde to collaborate on a project investigating patient adherence to treatment. Dr Smith expresses her concern that she was not approached for the permission to use the database. It had, after all, been set up with her grant money, which was continuing to provide training to the clinic's staff. However, in Dr Sekidde's view, the database constituted a donation to the clinic. He knew that the collaboration came with certain expectations, but felt that the clinic had more than compensated for this 'gift' by giving Dr Smith access to Dr Sekidde's 'valuable patients'.

QUESTIONS

- What makes Dr Sekidde feel uneasy about the collaboration? Are his anxieties justified?
- What about Dr Smith's concerns? In which ways is the database hers and in which ways is it not?
- What do you think the implications might be for Dr Sekidde if he collaborates with the Norwegian team? What do you think he should do?
- Should the Norwegian team have contacted Dr Smith first?
- Who owns the computerized database and who has the right to use it for research? Who has priority?
- In what ways are Dr Sekidde's patients valuable? For whom, and in what ways?
- What rights do the patients have with regard to their data?

- What does this story demonstrate about some of the advantages and disadvantages of international collaboration?
- What measures could have been taken to prevent conflict between the collaborators?

REFLECTION ON YOUR OWN EXPERIENCES

- In your own research setting, are there guidelines for data sharing and management?
- Whose interests do these guidelines protect?
- What are the advantages and disadvantages of formalizing plans for access to data and ownership of patient information? What are the pros and cons of more informal agreements?

ACTIVITY

Divide participants into small groups of four to six and ask them either to critique any existing guidelines for data sharing used at your institution, or to agree on key components of data-sharing agreements. Ask them to use the questions above to guide their discussions, and to consider the rights of patients concerning the use of their data in research.

FURTHER READING

Crane, J.T. (2011) Scrambling for Africa? Universities and global health. *The Lancet* 377(9775), 1388–1390.

Lang, T. (2011) Advancing global health research through digital technology and sharing data. *Science* 331(6018), 714–717.

Petryna, A. (2007) Clinical trials offshored: on private sector science and public health. *BioSocieties* 2(1), 21–40.

Ongoing consultations in the area of data sharing:
Bioethics, Research Ethics & Review. The ethics of data sharing. Available at: https://globalhealthreviewers.tghn.org/community/blogs/post/988/2013/11/the-ethics-of-data-sharing/ (accessed 25 October 2015).

BETWEEN ENVY, SUSPICION AND DESIRE:
EMBEDDING RESEARCH IN GOVERNMENT HEALTHCARE FACILITIES

FACILITATOR'S NOTES

This case study invites us to consider what can happen when research is embedded in regular state healthcare facilities. The story describes an intervention where extra equipment and staff training is provided to health facilities in the intervention arm of a trial. In addition to the trial, a sub-sample of children that attend the facility are followed closely to measure the impact of these additions on morbidity. In theory, anyone receiving services at the facilities in the intervention group should benefit from this research, as it should raise standards across the facility as a whole. In practice, however, children enrolled in the sub-study receive more attention than other patients, and receive travel reimbursements to reach the clinic. This special treatment distracts peoples' attention away from the wider efforts to improve the quality of care provided across the whole facility, and gives rise to envy.

Be careful to stress both the advantages and disadvantages of embedding research into routine healthcare settings, and encourage attendees to think about how to address some of the problems that can arise. As an example of a research project with multiple layers (a main intervention and a sub-study) this story is also helpful for thinking through the challenges of describing complex research.

LEARNING OBJECTIVE

To consider how research can change the landscape of healthcare provision, and to discuss how researchers can promote constructive collaboration with routine healthcare staff and local communities

KEYWORDS

Government

Standards of care

Inducements

Research versus care

BETWEEN ENVY, SUSPICION AND DESIRE:

EMBEDDING RESEARCH IN GOVERNMENT HEALTHCARE FACILITIES

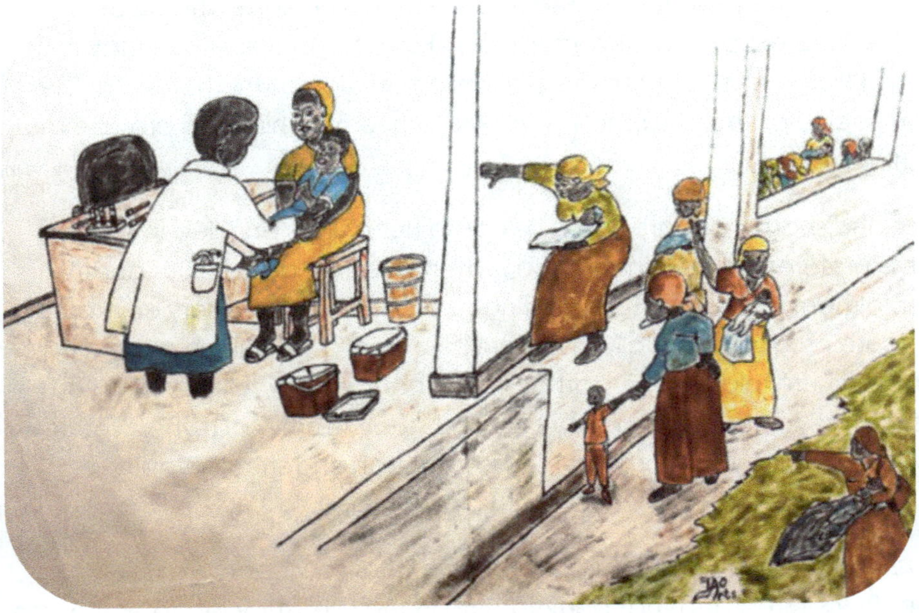

'WHY IS HER CHILD GETTING SPECIAL TREATMENT?'

THE STORY

A trial has taken place to improve the quality of services provided in lower-level government health facilities in a designated area. The intervention was funded by a Northern philanthropic foundation through a European university, collaborating with a major African teaching and referral hospital. In half of the area's health facilities, chosen by randomization, health workers were given extra training and the facilities were supplied with new diagnostic equipment. To test how well the project has worked, researchers compare comments from community members who attend the health facilities in the intervention arm with those who attend the facilities in the control group.

In addition, researchers randomly select a cohort of children from households across the area, to measure the impact of the project on disease. The children are periodically visited in their homes by members of the study team. They are also given a special card to present during their visits to the health centres, to record all treatments provided. For all such visits, the caregivers are provided with transport – either reimbursed in cash or picked up by the project car to get to and from the facility. The treatment records are collated as part of interviews conducted by fieldworkers in participants' homes. As a 'token of thanks', participants and their families are given sugar and tea on these occasions.

At the end of the study, a group discussion is called by the project's social scientists, to talk about patients' experiences of the project. This meeting is facilitated by two social scientists from the study team. Most of the people in the group say they have not noticed any improvements in the quality of the service at their health centre – even those who have been visiting clinics, which received the extra funding and training. But one participant, a lady in her early thirties, protests, stating that she always received excellent service at the health facility: 'For me, every time I visit I receive proper treatment – they examine my child and provide me with the required medication.'

The other participants jeer and sharply disagree: 'It is because her child is enrolled in this special group that she gets preferential treatment.' The lady in question agrees. But another participant argues that enrolment in the sub-study was no guarantee of good service. Rather, she has found that healthcare providers actually discriminate against the children who are enrolled in the special group. She explains: 'The staff at health centre, they tell you that you are just faking your illness so that you can get money from the study team. And when you try to explain the illness they tell you that you should not feel so special, and should stop telling them what to do'.

In the course of the discussion there appears to be a consensus that services have not improved in any of the health centres, and that participating in the sub-study led to one or the other form of discrimination by nurses in the centres – with the exception of the one discussant who expressed satisfaction.

Yet, despite the mainly negative comments about the treatment of children enrolled in the special study, and no one mentioning improvements in the intervention facilities, some of the participants raise some new questions as the discussion draws to a close: Why did the study team not visit their own village? Why hadn't they enrolled any children from their village? 'Ever since this study started, I have never seen any members of the study team in our village. Is it because they do not think we have problems, or what? Or is it because the study nurse prays together with the head mistress there?' Addressing the moderator directly, one person adds: 'Please tell your people that we also have problems in our village and we need your help.'

The social scientists end the meeting at a loss as to what to respond or what to tell their colleagues.

QUESTIONS

- What ethical and practical issues are raised by the somewhat contradictory positions expressed in this discussion?
- How do research activities alter the landscape of healthcare, and what ethical issues emerge from inclusion and exclusion in research projects?
- How can we explain the tension between suspicion and desire among research participants?
- How can we explain the reported behaviour of the health facility staff?
- How do you think this situation could be avoided or managed?

REFLECTION ON YOUR OWN EXPERIENCES

- From your experience, are research participants keen to enter new projects, or are they suspicious – or both? How are these emotions expressed?
- What different kinds of reactions and behaviours have you observed among healthcare personnel, when engaging with medical research projects?

FURTHER READING

Street, A. (2012) Affective infrastructure: hospital landscapes of hope and failure. *Space and Culture* 15(1), 44–56.

Sullivan, N. (2012) Enacting spaces of inequality: placing global/state governance within a Tanzanian hospital. *Space and Culture* 15(1), 57–67.

THE END OF A TRIAL:
POST-TRIAL RESPONSIBILITES AND RELATIONSHIPS

FACILITATOR'S NOTES

This case study raises difficult questions about the blurred lines between health research and medical care in places where access to routine healthcare is limited. In such settings, it is arguably unethical to conduct research without catering for study participants' general healthcare needs. But what are the appropriate boundaries for this care? For whom are researchers responsible, and for how long?

In this story, the research team agreed to a request from a village elder to extend the provision of free healthcare to all villagers, instead of just restricting it to study participants, and worked hard to establish a continuity of care for both participants and employees. This created a good rapport between the research programme and the community, and supported trial recruitment. Now, however, the research team leader faces a difficult situation: the trial has ended with no prospect of new research involving the same participants in the near future. This creates difficulties for both participants and staff, and might threaten other future projects. So how should research organizations prepare for such situations? How can they manage community expectations, and what can they do to mitigate negative effects?

There are no easy answers, but you could get participants to think about the advantages and disadvantages of researchers' working closely with routine healthcare providers; the need to make funders and research sponsors more aware of these challenges; and the need to be realistic and practical in managing community expectations.

LEARNING OBJECTIVE

To consider the problems of ending trials when research has become a major part of the healthcare landscape, and to identify solutions for managing these challenges

KEYWORDS

Post-trial care

Long-term engagement

Government

Standards of care

THE END OF THE TRIAL:
POST-TRIAL RESPONSIBILITIES AND RELATIONSHIPS

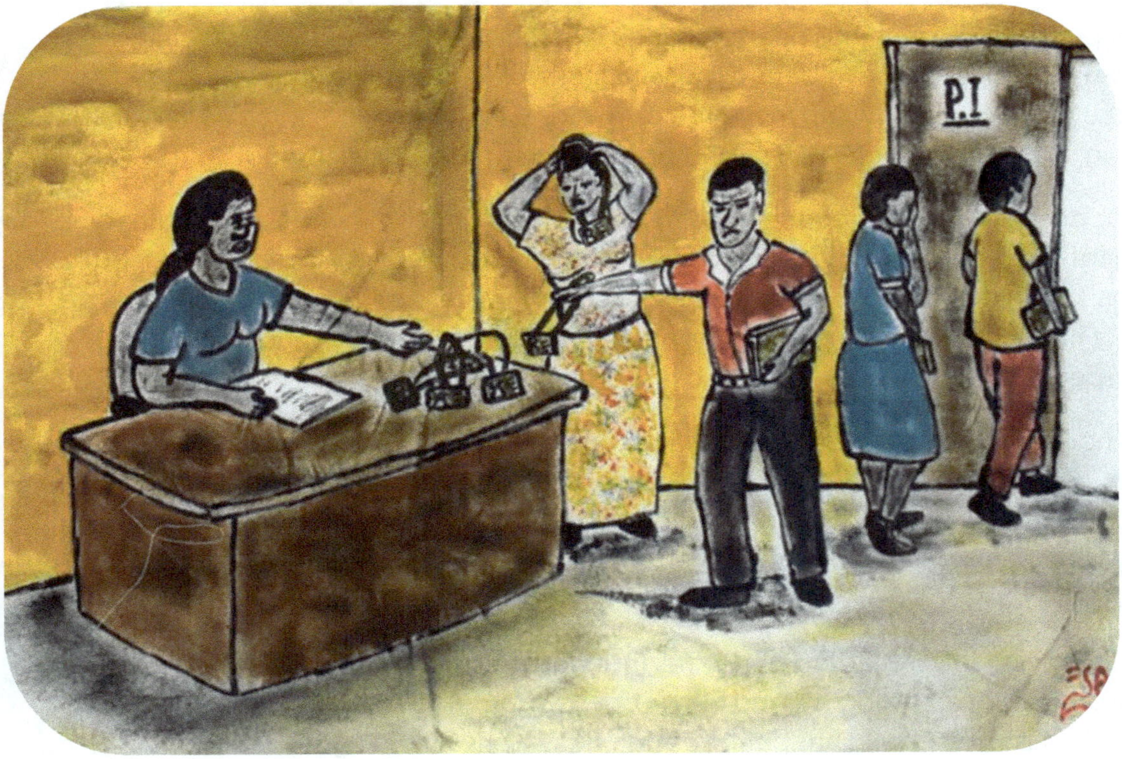

STAFF WERE NOT PLEASED TO RECEIVE THEIR END OF CONTRACT LETTERS

THE STORY

Akono, the trial coordinator of a large-scale three-year vaccine trial which is ending, has called a final staff meeting. It is two weeks since the last blood samples were collected, and it's essential to get everyone together before the staff leave for home for good. Sitting around a seminar table, he assures the 25 nurses, fieldworkers, and drivers that they will all be receiving reference letters from the trial, but that it is uncertain when a new research project might begin. It seems unlikely that he can retain most of the team on contract.

Privately, Akono is frustrated. In the past, the projects that he has managed have followed on from each other quickly, allowing him to re-hire and extend staff contracts. There are fieldworkers in this group that he has worked with for over ten years – workers who know the local communities, and are well known and accepted. The current gap after the end of this project means that if a new study starts, not only will he have to retrain a whole new group, but he'll also need to rebuild the trust this team has worked so hard to establish with the community. 'If it were up to me,' he tells the group, 'I would keep you all on staff. Unfortunately, it is not; funding decisions are outside of my scope. This is up to the donors and people up there. Does anyone have any questions?'

Ebrima, a project nurse who has been stationed in a remote village at the edge of the study area, raises his hand. 'We have been living with them for almost three years, sharing meals, taking care of their families when they are sick. We are giving them the vaccine and then we are leaving. They worked hard with us and we are letting them down. It is not right.'

Akono has anticipated these concerns. With nurses living with communities for months on end, a number of close connections and friendships have formed between staff and their patients. Ebrima, he knows, took his job very seriously, and many of the participants from that village spoke very highly of him and the quality of his care. 'Yes, I know they will not be happy,' Akono responds. 'But they knew this was a research project. It has a beginning and an end.'

Ebrima is not convinced. 'The station is still here and other projects will come in the future, perhaps even soon. We could continue working with them until the next one comes. At community level, it would help a great deal. If we leave just like that, the next time they will say "You people, we only see you when you want something from us and then we don't see you again."'

Akono is beginning to get irritated. He knows that bad community feelings could have serious repercussions for future research – and also for his own job success. To enrol the necessary numbers into this vaccine trial he spent weeks in discussions with village leaders, and worked hard to meet their demands. He even extended the provision of free healthcare from volunteers and their families to all residents within a participant village. A resentful nurse, especially one who has just lost his job, is exacerbating an already difficult meeting. 'Like you,' Akono replies abruptly, 'participants are on a contract. Your job now is over.'

As he leaves the meeting, Ebrima shakes his head. 'I don't know how they are going to tell them but it is going to be a big problem. We are from the same community and I will meet them, at festivals, in town. How can I look them in the eye?'

QUESTIONS

- What are Ebrima's main concerns? What are Akono's? And what are the research participants'?
- In which ways do these concerns overlap, and in which ways do they not?

- What do you think about Ebrima's suggestion? Is keeping a nurse posted in a study area after the end of a trial a good idea? Why, or why not? What about the practicalities?
- While funding decisions are beyond Akono's control, are there other things he could do to make things easier for staff and participants? How, and why, might the project planners support him in this?

REFLECTION ON YOUR OWN EXPERIENCES

- In your own research setting, what are the procedures when trials come to an end?
- How do local people understand the timeframe of research, and what are their expectations of the relationship with staff?
- How have you managed these expectations in the past? What are the risks – for participants and staff – of associating research with healthcare? What are the benefits?

FURTHER READING

Kelly, A.H., Pinder, M., Ameh, D., Majambere, S., and Lindsay, S. (2011) 'Like Sugar and Honey': the embedded ethics of a larval control project in The Gambia. *Social Science & Medicine* 70 (12), 1912–1919.

Lairumbi, G.M. et al. (2011) Ethics in practice: the state of the debate on promoting the social value of global health research in resource-poor settings, particularly Africa. *BMC Medical Ethics* 12(22), 1–8.

Will, C.M. (2011) Mutual benefit, added value? Doing research in the National Health Service. *Journal of Cultural Economy* 4(1), 11–26.

HELPING HAND:
WORKING WITH PUBLIC HOSPITALS

FACILITATOR'S NOTES

This case study describes the activities of a fieldworker who accompanies one of 'his' research participants through their treatment at a public hospital. The fieldworker wants to ensure that the participant receives the best possible treatment, but also to check that the data recorded is of the high quality needed to meet standards for reporting Serious Adverse Events (SAEs). In the process, this fieldworker experiences friction with hospital staff.

This is a common medical research situation. As well as raising questions about the different resources available to research staff and government health workers, the story suggests differences in how the two groups perceive each other and how their communication styles differ, and points to cultural, gender, and generational differences.

The group could be guided to distinguish between different levels of interactions in the story: the personal level (experienced by the fieldworker and hospital staff), the institutional level (the role of the research organization and the hospital), and the global level (the systemic resource gap between international research and national funding for healthcare). Possible solutions could emerge at any of these levels: changing personal styles of communication; more frequent engagement meetings and other shared activities between the hospital and researchers; or larger-scale structural interventions like long-term partnerships to address systemic inequality and improve hospital facilities.

Ideally, the discussion would move beyond Jonah's shortcomings as an individual, to consider institutional practices. This case invites practical solutions to improving

LEARNING OBJECTIVE

To explore different viewpoints and interests when government health facilities collaborate with transnational research bodies – and to explore the challenges facing individuals in an unequal system

KEYWORDS

Standards of care

Clinical responsibility

Government

Capacity building

Research versus care

communication and collaboration. The institutional practices in the study can be questioned: how was the research project introduced to healthcare personnel? What sort of agreement exists between the research programme and healthcare institution? Is this in writing, and accessible to staff? Does it specify particular practices and resources? How often do representatives and staff from the institutions meet, and at which level? What ownership does the hospital have in results and publications? Do hospital doctors receive any other benefits from the collaboration, such as training? What sorts of stereotypes exist with regard to the other group? The discussion could be guided towards improvements in any or all of these issues, perhaps through formal procedures, including complaints procedures on both sides.

HELPING HAND:
WORKING WITH PUBLIC HOSPITALS

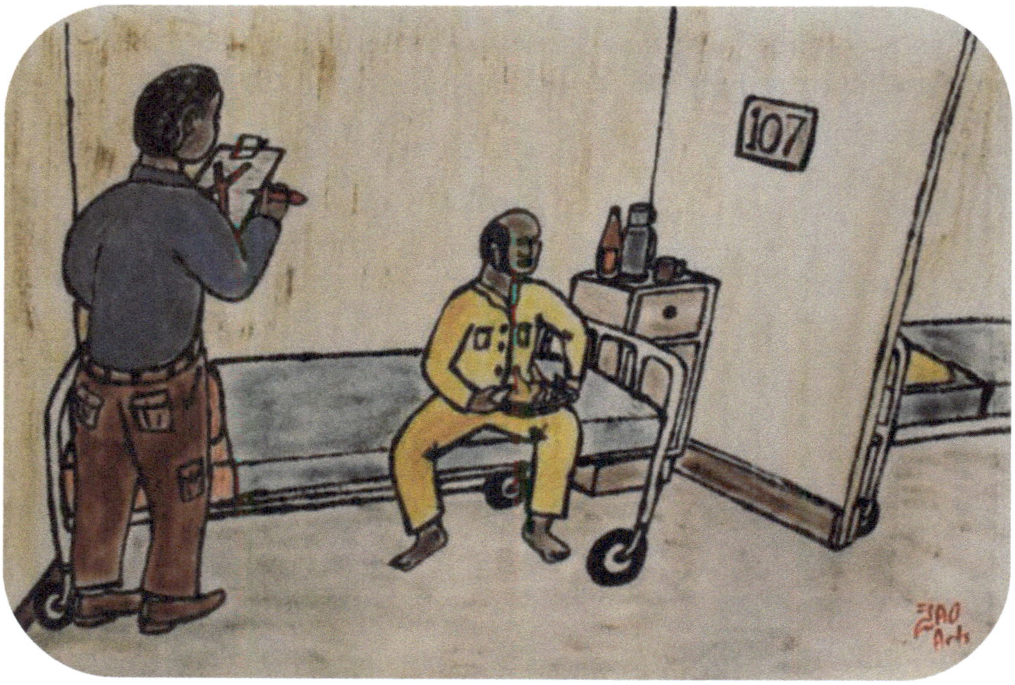

BARRABAS ATE THE CHICKEN JONAH HAD BROUGHT HIM, WHILE JONAH CHECKED HIS CHART FOR MISTAKES

THE STORY

A multi-country malaria vaccine trial, following good clinical practice and international trial regulations, monitors all adverse events, and offers full in- and out-patient care for participants throughout the project. Sick participants are referred for in-patient care to the national hospital, where the research clinic is hosted. Costs for hospitalization, laboratory and other procedures, and drugs, are paid for directly by the trial. This collaboration has been in place for several decades, but without a detailed written memorandum.

Barrabas, the oldest study participant, suffers from serious heart arrhythmia. Halfway through the trial his concerns worsen and he is admitted to the hospital. Jonah, a fieldworker who has become friendly with Barrabas after repeated home visits for data collection, visits him in the ward several times a day.

Jonah previously worked as a porter in the same public hospital and is familiar with hospital routines and procedures (as well as with their potential shortcomings). He begins each day by reading Barrabas' medical file. If he does not find the file by the bedside, he goes to the nurses in charge, whom he knows, and runs through the file with them.

Based on his on-the-job training as a fieldworker on this study, Jonah identifies gaps in both the treatment and the routine measurements that he needs for adverse event reporting. Today he sees that no respiratory rates were taken (or recorded); temperature values are missing; and it is not clear when the patient was last seen by the consultant. Jonah, who has been employed by the international research organization for several years, and has become very self-confident, scolds the young hospital nurse, and explains (in somewhat politer terms) to the matron of the ward that proper routines had not been observed – but not why it matters for the trial.

Jonah fills in some of the missing records himself after taking rates and measurements, and hands the file back to the clinician in charge who has arrived for his ward round. The clinician mentions that Barrabas' heart rates are a bit low and that an ECG is needed. Seeing that this is in the best interest of 'his' patient, Jonah immediately assures the doctor that the research project will pay for the ECG and insists that a written request is immediately prepared. Aware of the complicated procedures of queueing, appointment-making, and payment for such procedures, Jonah goes and pays the small fee to the hospital cashier, and takes Barrabas straight through to the ECG nurse. Just 20 minutes later they are back on the ward.

'This ECG alone would have taken a few days, if I had not been there,' Jonah comments to himself. 'How can we work with this hospital if they can't even take a pulse regularly? How can I fill my SAE form with this sort of data?'

When Jonah returns to the research clinic in a different building, the study coordinator tells him that he has had a call from the hospital, complaining about interference in clinical procedures. They both shrug it off as the sort of 'inevitable' friction which has to be 'endured' in order to procure adequate care and valid data.

After work that day, Jonah passes by the supermarket, and buys half a roast chicken to bring to Barrabas on the hospital ward. He noticed earlier that Barrabas has lost weight whilst in hospital. Jonah has now known Barrabas for two years. He has visited him at home, discussed personal problems with him, and assisted in his treatment on occasion. Visiting him in hospital, Jonah feels like he is not just visiting a research participant, but caring for a friend.

QUESTIONS

- Why is Jonah's intervention in the hospital setting relevant to the success of the research? How might it endanger it?

- What motivates Jonah's detailed investigation and engagement with Barrabas' care?
- What expertise does Jonah draw upon, and how did he come by it?
- What happens to the knowledge that Jonah brings to, and gains by, his work in helping Barrabas? What else might he have done with this knowledge – in relation to both the hospital, and the research team?
- What do you think about Jonah's relationship with the public hospital staff? What different factors shape this relationship?
- Why did the hospital doctor call and complain about Jonah's activity in the hospital? Could the doctor have done something else? What do you think about the reaction of Jonah and the study coordinator? Do you think such friction is 'inevitable' and must just be 'endured'? Why do you think Jonah and his colleague view it this way?
- How might knowledge of the way the local hospital works impact the *findings* of the research? Do you think this is helpful? What changes could be made in referral policies for the trial?
- What might be done, at what levels, to avoid the situation repeating itself? (The facilitator's notes have some suggestions.)
- What do you think individuals can do when facing structural inequalities in healthcare?

ACTIVITY

Put yourself in Jonah's shoes. What would your reaction be to the shortcomings of the hospital's routines and provisions? What would you do about them? What care would you have to take when doing so? Then take the opposite perspective, of the different members of staff in the public hospital. How do they each perceive Jonah? How might they react next time?

REFLECTION ON YOUR OWN EXPERIENCES

- Can you think of contexts where research staff or clinicians at your workplace draw upon specific local knowledge or informal contacts in order to help research?
- Are there similar situations where knowledge of your local health system is necessary in order to 'make ends meet' and facilitate successful collaboration?
- How far should a research project go in addressing the shortcomings of local healthcare provision? What are the challenges of this?
- Are there times when you have felt helpless in the face of global-level inequality? If so, how have you responded?

FURTHER READING

Chantler, T., Otewa, F. et al. (2013) Ethical challenges that arise at the community interface of health research: village reporters' experiences in Western Kenya. *Developing World Bioethics* 13(1), 30–37.

Street, A. (2012) Affective infrastructure: hospital landscapes of hope and failure. *Space and Culture* 15(1), 44–56.

Sullivan, N. (2012) Enacting spaces of inequality: placing global/state governance within a Tanzanian hospital. *Space and Culture* 15(1), 57–67.

Whyte, S. R. (2014) Therapeutic research in low-income countries: studying trial communities. *Archives of Disease in Childhood* 99(11), 1029 -1032.

WHOSE CAPACITY?: COLLABORATION THROUGH CAPACITY BUILDING

FACILITATOR'S NOTES

Capacity building in the South is one of the key aspirations of collaborations in transnational biomedical research, especially in partnerships involving researchers and institutions from the North. Collaborations have been hailed as beneficial to all involved, and many collaborative agreements have capacity building as one of the core objectives and an indicator of good collaboration. Although the general consensus among African research scientists is that collaborations are good and must be encouraged, some disquiet is emerging regarding the actual benefits that emerge in different collaborative arrangements.

This case study invites us to think about a range of issues which emerge within collaborations, especially between unequal partners. Most North-South collaborations involve the transfer of a substantial amount of resources (funds, technical expertise and organization) to the African institution, in exchange for access to desired patient populations and expert colleagues who can shepherd proposals through local ethical review. Collaborations imply equality, but can there be equality between unequal partners? This case study asks us to consider whether collaboration as a paradigm serves to create the desired equality or, rather, hinders open discussions of the same. Should collaborating partners strive for more 'equitable' collaborations, or change the entire paradigm?

LEARNING OBJECTIVE

To consider the nature of scientific collaborations and the rhetoric of equality between Northern and Southern partners, especially around questions of capacity building of both human expertise and infrastructure

KEYWORDS

Capacity building

North-South relationships

WHOSE CAPACITY?:
COLLABORATION THROUGH CAPACITY BUILDING

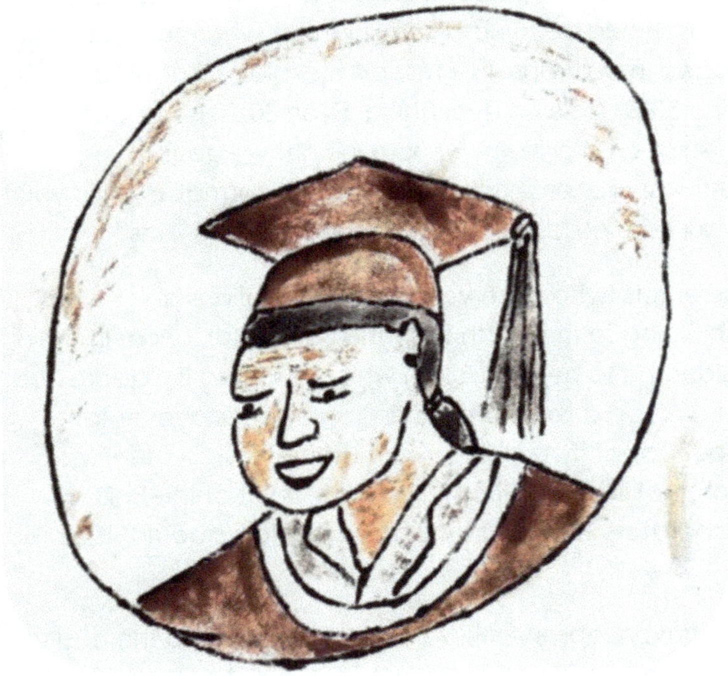

LUCY WAS PLEASED SHE HAD GOT HER CHANCE, BUT THE ISSUE OF SPONSORSHIP WAS A THORNY ONE

THE STORY

A group of African scientists are having a discussion over drinks in a pub, after a workshop on the role of collaboration in capacity building in their institutions. In their stories and experiences, various differing views emerge about the prospect, nature and outcome of capacity building initiatives in Africa. Through their different stories, told with lots of humour and laughter, three differing propositions emerge.

Timothy, a senior scientist at an African national research institute, has this to say about collaborations and capacity building: 'Collaborations are very good, because from them we are able to develop both the human and infrastructural capacity of our institutions. Everything you see in my institution here, which by the way is exemplary, has been acquired through collaborations. And if it were not for collaborations, the director and I would not be professors at the moment. In terms of relationships with our collaborators from the North, we are their equals. We are even allowed to be Principal Investigators in projects initiated by them.'

Musa, another scientist, however, disagrees. He counters that in reality collaborations may not be as equal as presented by his colleague. He argues that collaborations are by their very nature unequal and imbalanced. 'You know us scientists! We "collaborate" in full knowledge of this inequality, and we are content with the little we get. Otherwise, we would stand to lose even this little support if we insisted on an equal share of everything.' The group of scientists who support his position in this discussion maintain that the collaborations they are involved in have resulted in capacity building in favour of the North, but this does not bother them. They consider this to be normal – the way things should be. One of the scientists who manages a very successful research institution engaged in collaborative research explains it candidly: 'Collaborations do not necessarily imply a 50:50 stake in everything. Even 80:20 is acceptable. For example, when we have ten scholarships on a project, we know eight will go to candidates from our collaborator's country, while we shall get two. That is normal. Even in your own family, you must first take care of your own children before your neighbours' kids.'

A third position is put forward by other scientists, who observe that collaborations as constituted do provide more capacity building to the North than the South. But, unlike in their colleagues above, these scientists consider this to be a problem which ought to be addressed. One of the scientists, who has worked in collaborative research engagements for over ten years, has this to say: 'When we talk about capacity building, we must now ask, whose capacity? You find nowadays when a project is funded from the North, most of the PhD students employed come from our collaborators in the North. Can we still talk about this as capacity building to the South?'

Lucy, who is a research director in her institution, observes: 'We have now come to the end of a very long collaborative research programme which has been on for the last 14 years, and we are doing our reviews of the project. And to our astonishment, we have realized that human capacity building has been tilted in favour of the North. Most of those we have trained over the last 14 years have been students from the North – yet the whole programme was billed as capacity building initiative for Africa. This cannot be right. We need to do something new'.

QUESTIONS:

- The three groups of scientists disagree with each other about both the nature of North-South collaboration and whether or not it should be changed. Which view do you think best sums up North-South collaborations? Why?
- Why do you think Timothy, Musa and Lucy have different perspectives on collaboration?
- Musa uses an analogy of a family 'feeding their children first' to justify unequal resource allocation between partners in terms of funding PhD scholarships. Do you agree or

disagree with this analogy, and why? What do you think the long-term consequences of such practices could be for both North and South partners?

- This story only focuses on the opinion of the South partners. What do you imagine their Northern counterparts might say about collaboration? Do you think they would share the views of Timothy, Musa, or Lucy?

- Lucy says, 'We need to do something new.' What kind of 'new' collaboration practices can you imagine? How would you like the future of collaboration to look? What barriers do you think might need to be overcome to reach this goal?

- Short of changing global inequalities, are there any immediate, practical steps that could be put in place to create better collaborations?

REFLECTIONS ON YOUR OWN EXPERIENCE:

- How would you describe the type of collaboration your institution has with its partners? (For example, 'contented'? 'Equal'? 'Awkward'?)

- How do you feel about this collaboration? Does your perspective fit one of the three views described above or do you have another, different, view?

- What are the strengths and weakness of the collaborations of your institution?

- How do you think your institution's collaborations could be improved? What are the barriers to this? Can you offer realistic solutions to how they can be overcome?

- Has your institution faced a situation where collaboration has broken down? What happened? Why? What could have been done differently?

FURTHER READING

Chu, K.M., Jayaraman, S., Kyamanywa, P., Ntakiyiruta, G. (2014) Building research capacity in Africa: equity and global health collaborations. *PloS Med* 11(3), e1001612.

Jentsch, B. and Pilley C. (2003) Research relationships between the South and the North: Cinderella and the ugly sisters? *Social Science and Medicine* 57, 1957–1967.

Panitch, V. (2013) Exploitation, justice, and parity in international clinical research. *Journal of Applied Philosophy* 30(4), 304–31

LIKE A MARKET:
COMPETITIVE RECRUITMENT AND DOUBLE ENROLMENT

FACILITATOR'S NOTES

This case study is about recruitment procedures for two new research projects, what participants do in order to secure a place on a trial, and how researchers try to balance recruitment targets with study protocols and ethical standards. It also raises questions about collaboration between different research organizations operating in the same area, and the confidentiality of participants' data.

One key issue that this case highlights are the different material and immaterial interests which are important to different stakeholders, and how these shape practices. For example, the researchers have to change their recruitment practices in order to demonstrate their competence and maintain their reputation. Another issue arising from this is how these interests and practices might conflict or agree with fundamental ethical principles.

LEARNING OBJECTIVE

To reflect upon the challenges of institutional coordination, participant inducement, and competitive recruitment in intensely studied geographic areas, and to consider the role of research participation as a valuable resource for both researchers and participants

KEYWORDS

Inducements

Recruitment

Money

LIKE A MARKET:
COMPETITIVE RECRUITMENT AND DOUBLE ENROLMENT

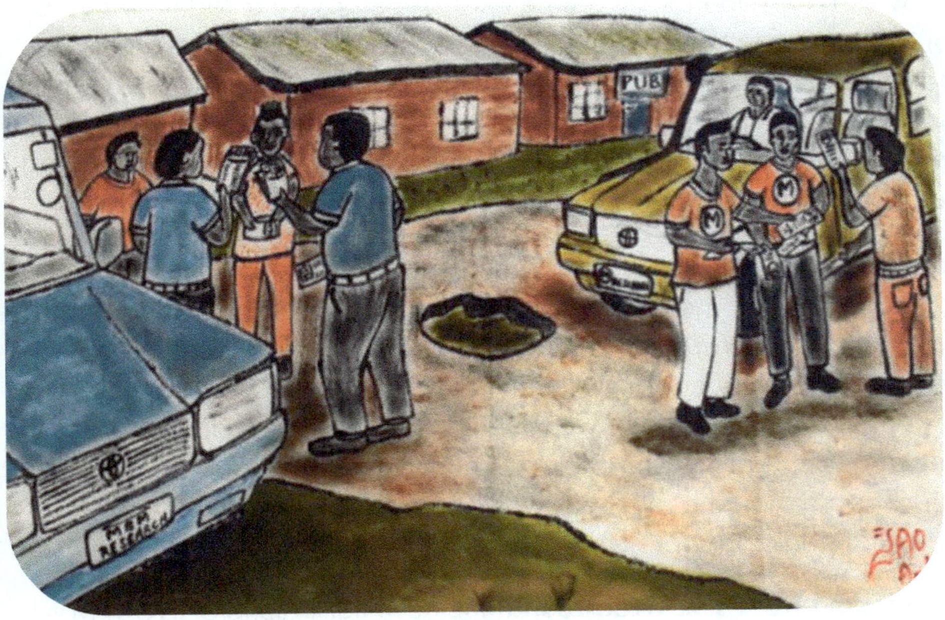

'SUDDENLY EVERYONE WANTS TO KNOW US!'

THE STORY

A multi-site trial of treatment-as-prevention (TAP) for HIV, conducted by an international consortium, tests the efficacy of new drugs. Participants on this trial have to be sexually active, HIV negative men-having-sex-with-men (MSM).

Due to the massive stigma (and national legislation) against homosexuality, this type of research participant is in limited supply, and the researchers working in each location have to go outside their usual areas to find enough people. There is a particular pressure to recruit participants quickly, because the international consortium has directed each site to find a set number before a certain date, so nearby projects will have to compete for those who could join either study. The more participants each site can recruit, the more it can contribute to the overall sample, and thereby increase its share in the overall findings and its reputation.

To make things more complicated, similar participants are needed by other HIV prevention research projects in the area. Young, HIV negative male participants who have sex with men are in high demand – partly because of their high infection risk, and partly because this target group has recently gained a high profile globally, so there is lots of funding to reach them. Normally, each research organization operates in different rural districts. However, the new interest in MSM, and the pressure for high recruitment rates, leads two particular organizations to step into each other's 'territory' in recruiting men from the whole region.

These two organizations, which both operate in remote rural areas, have worked together to agree standard rates of 'transport reimbursement' for participants. These rates are usually based on protocols and consent forms. The ongoing HIV prevention trials, however, complicate this arrangement, partly because it requires people to travel much larger distances, needing larger, staggered reimbursements of travel cost. Therefore, reimbursement conditions are adjusted over the course of the trial.

As a lead scientist privately admits regarding these payments, it is very important 'not to fall behind what the other group is offering the participants' in terms of transport reimbursement and other benefits such as lunches during clinic visits, so as not to lose out on recruitment. As he is well aware, 'participants hear about many trials, and shop around and compare, it's like a market' – so one has to know what the others are doing. He cites several occasions when participants at public information meetings about the trial have asked for improved benefits, referring to what (they had heard that) the other trial was providing. 'And yet,' he adds, 'we do not want to end up paying participants.'

Participants who consider themselves as MSM realize that this new trial, in spite of its awkward conditions, including coital diaries and regular physical examinations, entails particular benefits. These are not all material. People in this group are keen to learn more about the risk of HIV and possibilities to reduce it, and also, not insignificantly, are keen to meet people sharing similar problems. The confidential recruitment phone line is busy responding to large numbers of young men seeking to enrol. Staff who work on participant travel discuss reports that people are so keen that they travel over 100 miles, pretending to be residents of the wider study area, in order to take part.

Staff also wonder whether actually all the men involved in this trial really do have sex with men, and surmise that some of the participants have registered for more than one trial simultaneously. Such double enrolment can have a serious negative impact on the health of the participants, and the ethics and validity of the research. Responding to these suspicions, staff from different research organizations meet, compare records, and identify several men participating in both trials – in some cases even using different names. In response to this severe medical, ethical and scientific challenge, the research organizations agree to jointly finance a costly joint biometric database, in order to prevent future double enrolment.

QUESTIONS

- What are the key ethical issues at stake here? Try to identify several, related to very different areas of ethical consideration.
- What are the risks of the pressure to recruit participants, and for whom?
- What solutions could the research organizations try, in response to the pressures of competitive recruitment, and the other challenges of operating within the same region and population?
- What 'immaterial benefits' do you think the research offers participants (including those who have lied in order to take part)?
- What happens to informed consent, if participants are so keen to join the trial and work so hard to fit the criteria? Is the trial genuinely 'voluntary' now? What could project planners do about this?
- Do you think it is realistic that most ethics guidelines insist that the flow of resources, medicines, specimens, and information in research is non-economic? Do you think this reflects reality on the ground? If not, how could guidelines be amended, or what should be done in order to reflect real-life experience whilst also ensuring that research is not exploitative?

ACTIVITY

- Try to write a short summary of standard operating procedures for recruitment, consent and data handling for an imaginary HIV prevention study. Then compare these procedures to the practices described in the story. What differences are there?
- Based on the scenario in the case study, form three groups of equal size: trial staff including local Principal Investigators, monitors from the overseas consortium, and local research participants and the community. What does each of these groups make of the solutions described above? First, discuss this briefly in each group, then debate it between the groups.

REFLECTION ON YOUR OWN EXPERIENCES

- Have you ever experienced pressure to recruit participants? How was this pressure made clear to you? Discuss with others how this is felt by different people at different levels within your organization.

? Have you encountered populations who are very keen to be recruited into a particular trial, or research in general? Have you observed people striving to meet inclusion criteria, or even adapting to them? How did you cope with this challenge?

FURTHER READING

Caulfield, T. (2005) Legal and ethical issues associated with patient recruitment in clinical trials: the case of competitive enrolment. *Health Law Review* 13(2–3), 58–61.

Kamuya, D., Marsh, V., and Molyneux, S. (2011) What we learned about voluntariness and consent: incorporating 'background situations' and understanding into analyses. *The American Journal of Bioethics* 11(8), 31–13. *PubMed PMID*: 21806436.

Simon, C. and Mosavel, M. (2010) Community members as recruiters of human subjects: ethical considerations. *American Journal of Bioethics* 10(3), 3–11.

UNDER ONE ROOF:
SHARING RESOURCES IN A DISTRICT HOSPITAL

FACILITATOR'S NOTES

The main aim of this case study is to generate discussion about sharing resources when conducting research. It raises questions about how this should be regulated, who should be responsible for case-by-case decision-making, and how those responsible can be supported.

It could be argued that the research leadership needs to support research nurses and doctors to act in accord with the Hippocratic Oath, and their professional codes of practice. This could imply that, when the same staff will be caring for patients who are both in a study and outside it, research budgets should extend to covering at least some of the costs of caring for those who are not within the study. On the other hand, should researchers have to assume responsibility for the failings of routine medical services to provide essential care?

Or should research only take place in settings where there will not be obvious differences in access to resources and standards of caregiving?

Or should health researchers assume an advocacy role in terms of quality of care, supporting patients and providers to lobby for improved healthcare structures, processes and outcomes? If yes, what effects (negative and positive) could this have in terms of the implementation of research?

LEARNING OBJECTIVE

To consider the challenges of conducting health research in resource-limited health facilities, where differences in care-giving between research and routine services can result in dilemmas about equitable access to resources and expertise

KEYWORDS

Clinical responsibility

Standards of care

Government

Capacity building

UNDER ONE ROOF:
SHARING RESOURCES IN A DISTRICT HOSPITAL

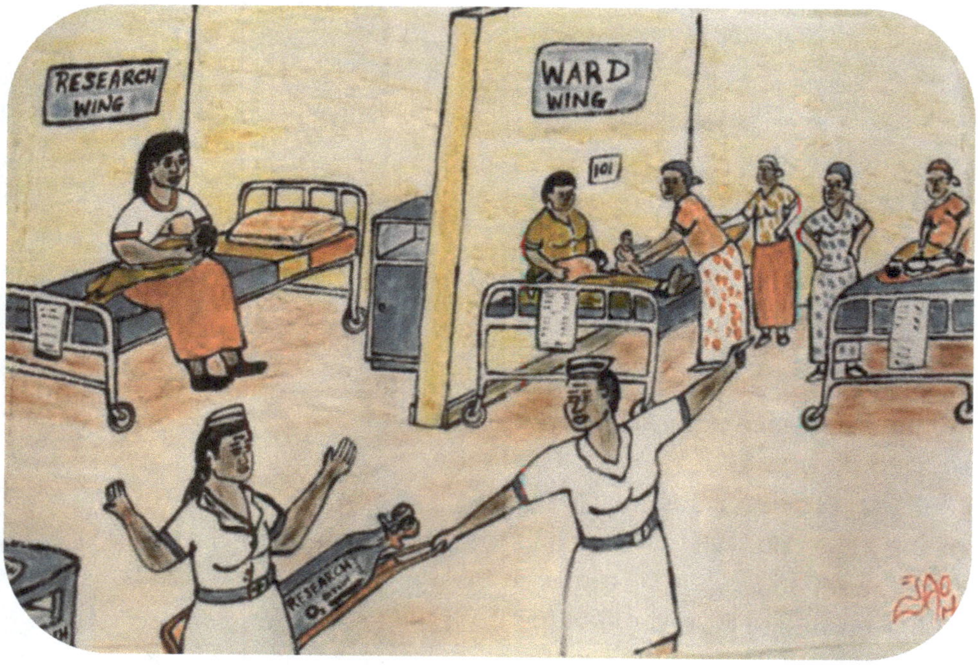

AS THEY BATTLED OVER THE OXYGEN, BEATRICE WONDERED WHAT THEY WERE FIGHTING FOR

THE STORY

Beatrice is a senior research nurse employed by a national health research organization, which collaborates with international researchers and medical research sponsors. She oversees the nursing care of paediatric study participants who become sick in the course of clinical trials taking place at a rural district hospital.

Trial participants are recruited in buildings adjacent to the hospital's main outpatient clinics. The hospital management board and medical superintendent have agreed to host trials, and entered into a memorandum of understanding (MOU) with the national research organization, which receives funding from international sponsors. The MOU outlines the points of agreement between the hospital and the research organization with regard to rent, use of hospital resources (space, water, electricity), and roles in patient care. Despite the hospital management's requests, however, there are no provisions for infrastructural improvements, as the international sponsor's funding regulations do not allow them to use funds to build lasting infrastructure.

The paediatric ward where Beatrice works has 30 beds in total, often occupied by more than one patient. She and her team of three research nurses are based in a separate bay on this ward, containing six beds. Research clinicians (including a fully qualified paediatrician) review the sick trial participants in this separate bay regularly. Other patients on the ward are cared for by four hospital nurses, three auxiliaries, and two hospital interns (recent medical school graduates) who are also responsible for various other wards.

Beatrice has quite a good relationship with the other ward nurses but they regularly ask to 'borrow' cannula and other resources allocated to the research patients, as hospital supplies run short on a regular basis. Beatrice and her team have access to separate nursing supplies, and the research doctors have access to a well-stocked formulary.

In the spirit of collaboration Beatrice is happy to share small items such as cannula, but less sure about medication. She talks to the trial coordinator and Principal Investigator about this and they meet with the ward staff and the medical superintendent to discuss how to move forward. They agree to share cheaper resources like analgesics fairly liberally, setting aside a budget to keep these in stock. But more expensive medications can only be given out in situations of emergency or particular need, on a case-to-case basis which will be judged by the trial paediatrician.

They also agree with the hospital to take turns in paying for oxygen cylinders to be refilled, to ensure a ready supply is available for all sick patients. The latter arrangement works for a month, until the hospital has another shortfall of funds. The research organization foots the bill for oxygen refills for a while, but then decides they will purchase their own oxygen cylinders and pay to refill them separately. They are under pressure from research sponsors to keep within the budget allocated to the research projects running at the district hospital.

Soon after that Beatrice receives a call from a junior nurse on night duty. The nurse tells her that an infant with severe pneumonia has been admitted to the ward and the hospital nurses need to 'borrow' the research oxygen cylinder in order to save the child. Beatrice is in two minds and does not know what to advise.

QUESTIONS:

- What are the key ethical issues at stake in this situation? Describe the challenges that this hospital-based research setting raises.
- What would you do if you were Beatrice? Would you follow the new regulations, or let the hospital nurses use the oxygen cylinder?
- What is the purpose of a Memorandum of Understanding (MOU) in these types of research collaborations, and what details should a MOU include?

- When research takes place in resource-limited health facilities, should research sponsors contribute financially to the care of patients who are not enrolled in research studies?

- Should research take place in settings where it is difficult for hospital staff to provide the same standards of care for both research and routine patients? Would it be better for research participants to be looked after in a separate ward? Should this ward be within the hospital environment or in a separate research facility? What would be the advantages and disadvantages of this, for patients and staff?

REFLECTION ON YOUR OWN EXPERIENCES

- Have you any experience with hospital-based research, or with using public health facilities in research?

- Have you ever been in a similar position to Beatrice? Share your experience, and explain what you did and why.

- How feasible do you think it is to regulate such resource-sharing arrangements? Who should draw these up, and how should practitioners be supported to follow them?

- How are project budgets drawn up in your place of work? Is allowance made for sharing resources?

FURTHER READING

Benatar, S.R. and Singer, P.A. (2010) Responsibilities in international research: a new look revisited. *Journal of Medical Ethics* 36(4), 194–197.

Brown, H. (2015) Global health partnerships, governance, and sovereign responsibility in western Kenya. *American Ethnologist* 42, 340–355. doi:10.1111/amet.12134

Street, A. (2014) Research in the clinic. In: Street, A. *Biomedicine in an Unstable Place: Infrastructure and Personhood in a Papua New Guinean hospital.* Duke University Press, Durham, North Carolina, 194–222.

WE WILL NOT DO YOUR WORK FOR FREE: INCENTIVES, PER DIEMS AND PROFESSIONAL CULTURE

FACILITATOR'S NOTES

The purpose of this case study is to encourage us to think critically about the use of per diems – especially in research which focuses on improving the quality of care, and does not directly involve patients. The participants in the story outlined below are healthcare workers who are required to make a change in their clinical practice for the purpose of a research project. This change involves some extra work, and although they are offered training and new skills in reward, they also request payment.

In effect, the healthcare workers do not believe that the intervention brings its own rewards. The researchers, however, believe that the study is just part of their existing professional duties, simply raising these to a new level, so no further incentive is required. This argument falls on deaf ears, however, partly due to the pervasive use of per diems elsewhere in medical research.

In your discussions, try to get participants to think critically about accepted practice, in order to develop objective arguments for or against the use of per diems in such instances.

LEARNING OBJECTIVE

To consider the advantages and disadvantages of using per diem payments in research, especially in research focusing on the quality of care rather than on new medical technologies

KEYWORDS

Standards of care

Government

Money

Capacity building

WE WILL NOT DO YOUR WORK FOR FREE:

INCENTIVES, PER DIEMS AND PROFESSIONAL CULTURE

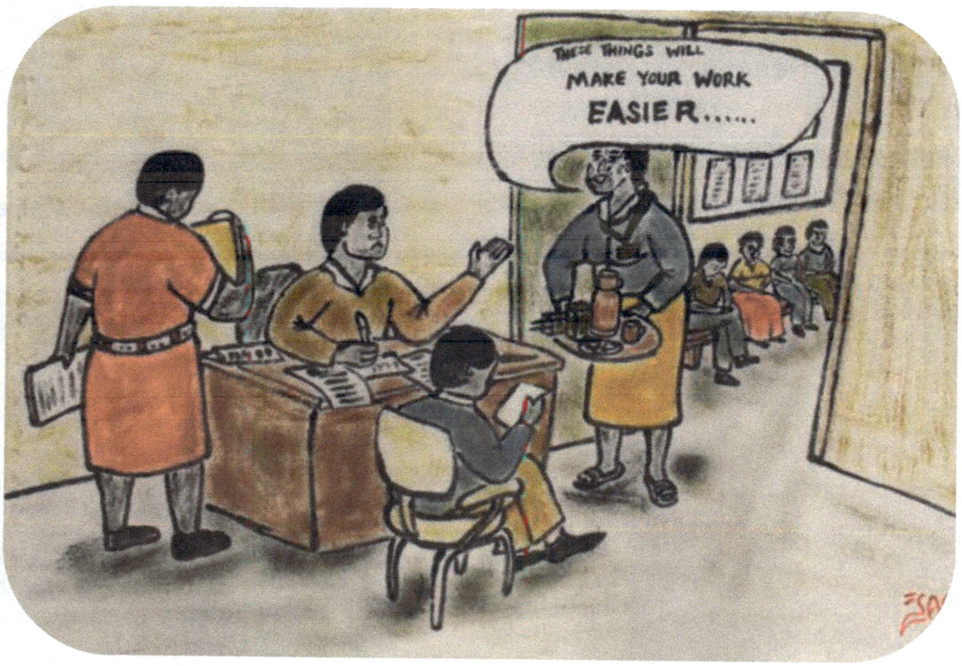

'THANK YOU FOR THE TEA BUT WHERE IS OUR PAYMENT...?'

THE STORY

A trial is being conducted to improve the quality of health services in lower-level government facilities in an African rural district. This involves retraining healthcare providers, and equipping them with skills to help them provide better care for their patients and to become better managers. This mostly involves reminding them of skills they learned in nursing and medical school, such as diagnosis and consultation skills for various medical conditions. However, some aspects, such as the use of new diagnostic equipment, are new to many of the participants. As well as these new practices, the intervention requires the healthcare workers to fill out four new columns in patients' records in the regular outpatient department register.

Most of the care providers participating acknowledge that the retraining and new tools make them better at their jobs, and help them look more professional in the eyes of their clients. They complain, however, that the 'retraining' takes too long, and that the new systems increase their workload and lead to delays in caring for patients.

The project's overseas Principal Investigators are determined not to pay per diems for the activities. According to them, the project falls under participants' routine duties; if anything, they should be grateful that the project retrains them and improves their skills for free. For their part, however, the participants consider the new duties involved in the trial as 'project work', over and above their ordinary tasks.

For this, they expect to be 'motivated'. They also state that extra columns in the registers 'consume too much of our ink' and that they are 'running out of ball pens' because of this. In response, the project team provide two pens per month for each of the workers, and asks them to report to the project coordinators any time they run out of pens. The health workers then complain that the workload is too heavy, and that they are spending all the day in the facility without a lunch break. The project team respond by buying them sugar, tea leaves and biscuits to make tea during their work.

Several weeks later the project team discovers that workers in some health centres are not carrying out most of the trial activities. They send one of the senior project leaders, a local medical doctor, to find out what is going on. When he arrives, the health workers inform him that their informed consent agreement allows them to withdraw from the project at any time, and that they are not required to give any reasons for their withdrawal. The project team therefore has no right to ask them to explain themselves. When pressed further to explain their reason, the workers declare that they will not 'work for free' for the project. They cite their experience with other projects where they were paid a per diem for any activity, even if the activity did not take long, and reiterate that they expect to be 'motivated' or they will not participate.

The project team maintains that they will not pay a per diem, and sends other high-ranking Ministry of Health officials to implore the health workers to participate in the project. Meanwhile, over 15 other research projects are taking place locally at the same time, all organized by different institutions and all requiring the services of healthcare providers. Most of these institutions 'motivate' participants for taking part in the projects.

QUESTIONS

- Why do you think that the research Principal Investigators did not want to pay per diems? What beliefs do they seem to have? Do you think they are right?
- Can you sympathize with the healthcare providers' position? Why?
- What do you think about how both sides addressed the challenge? Do you think the study team understood what was behind the participants' requests, or not? Why? What do you think each side could have done differently?
- What do you think about the use of per diems in this kind of research? Is there a difference between reimbursing participants in clinical trials, and those in service improvement studies? What, if any, are the differences between projects like this one, and ones which conduct other kinds of research?
- Can you think of other ways of motivating staff to support the research?
- If you were the study coordinators, what would you do next?

REFLECTION ON YOUR OWN EXPERIENCES

- Present the case for or against reimbursing the healthcare workers for carrying out the study intervention.
- Have you encountered similar situations in your work? What were these and how did you deal with them?

FURTHER READING

Conteh, L. and Kingori, P. (2010) Per diems in Africa: a counter-argument. *Tropical Medicine & International Health* 15(12), 1553–1555.

Ridde, V. (2010) Per diems undermine health interventions systems and research in Africa: burying our heads in the sand. *Tropical Medicine and International Health*. Doi.10.1111/j.1365-3156.2010.02607.x

Vian, T., Miller, C., Themba, Z., and Bukuluki, P. (2012) Perceptions of per diems in the health sector: evidence and implications. *Health Policy and Planning*, 10(1093), 1–10.

IS IT A GIFT, REALLY?: DRUG DONATIONS, ACCESS AND SOCIAL BENEFIT

FACILITATOR'S NOTES

This story explores questions about the local benefits of transnational drug donations and related research. It presents the case of a donation programme which includes phase 4 post-licensure evaluation activities for a new drug, aimed at providing information about long-term and rare side-effects. The drug being donated is an expensive, newly-licensed treatment aimed at preventing heart disease. Its current market price means that it is unlikely to be adopted as a recommended routine medication, or have any significant market, among the population where the programme takes place. Instead, the results of the evaluation are likely to increase the drug's market share in high-income populations, mainly in the global North. Yet, in the short term, the donation programme provides substantial benefits to patients and doctors in the recipient population.

Critics of the donation programme argue that it is a for-profit trial posing as charity. They are concerned that a vulnerable population is providing information for the longer-term benefit of wealthy patients elsewhere. Local clinicians, however, highlight the advantages of the programme for their patients – even if these are only temporary.

This case study is designed to trigger reflections on the relative social benefit of experimental interventions. In some cases, this is straightforward. For example, if a trial involves risky experimentation on vulnerable volunteers, with the aim of developing a drug targeted mainly at high-income populations –for example, testing anti-obesity drugs in malnourished populations – this is obviously problematic. If, at the other end of the scale, a trial tests, for example, a low-cost alternative to imported ultrasound examination gel, produced

LEARNING OBJECTIVE

To consider the challenges and benefits of drug research projects that have few (but sometimes significant) local benefits

KEYWORDS

Drug donation

Pharmaceutical industry

Standards of care

Long-term engagement

Media relations

by local doctors and scientists, this seems much less problematic. Most cases, however, are less clear-cut, and require careful and detailed assessment of the potential benefits and disadvantages. This type of careful analysis might result in the conclusion that whilst a particular intervention makes unjust use of vulnerable study participants, it is also beneficial in some ways for these participants and other actors. The tension between knowing that something is unfair, for oneself or others, and yet feeling compelled to go along with it, is one of the most interesting aspects of this case study, as it relates to wider questions of ethical deliberation and personal conscience.

This case encourages policymakers, researchers, study managers, and field staff to consider the social and long-term benefits of donation programmes carefully, and weigh these against immediate benefits. As researchers, we need to be keenly aware that our activities can be exploitative and can reinforce pre-existing injustices. We therefore we need to be careful that we do our best to address these health inequalities, rather than aggravate them.

As part of the group activity exploring the benefits and disadvantages of this particular programme, training participants should think carefully about larger and smaller benefits to different actors, such as patients, relatives or healthcare personnel. For example, a clinic head might receive income from a trial; a district doctor or nurse might find her work eased by the availability of drugs and other tools; a family caretaker might be relieved of the high costs of a less efficient, locally available drug; and patients may be able be able to prevent heart disease. A journalist or activist, on the other hand, might look to the wider context, relating the programme to wider discussions about multinational pharmaceutical companies, drug pricing, constraints on health systems, and global health inequalities. The discussion should explore the way these different levels of interest and engagement overlap.

IS IT A GIFT, REALLY?:

DRUG DONATIONS, ACCESS AND SOCIAL BENEFIT

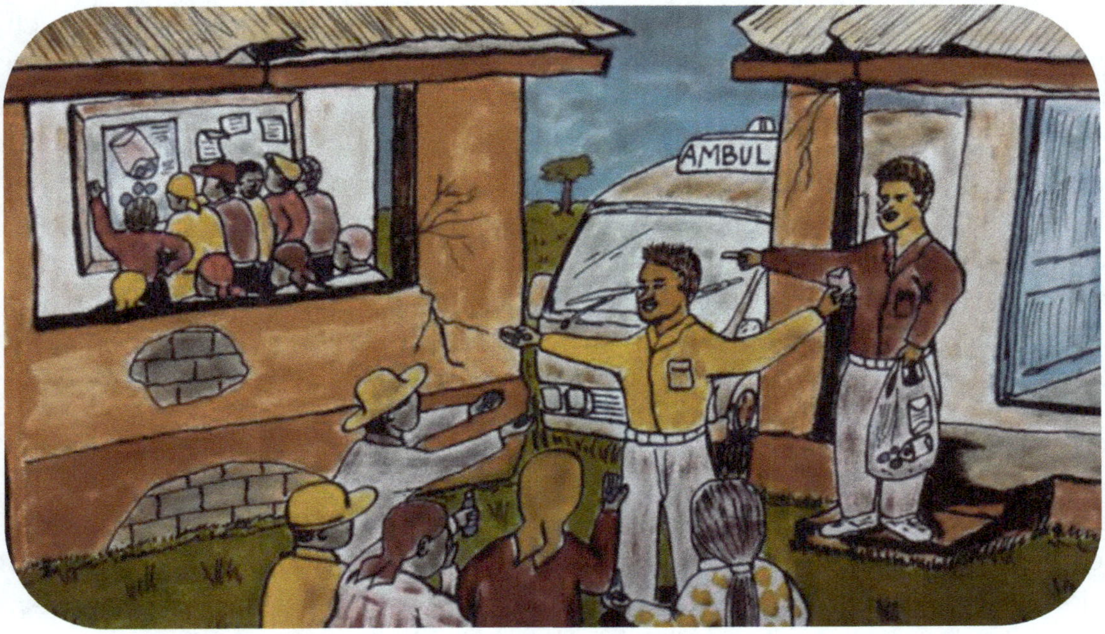

'THERE IS A NEW DRUG IN TOWN. IT'S FREE AND IT'S GOOD FOR YOUR HEART!'

THE STORY

X-22 is a novel prophylactic drug to prevent coronary heart disease. It has recently been licensed for use in North America and Europe, and is available in upmarket pharmacies in most African countries. But due to its cost of approximately US$90 per month, it is not widely used and there are no plans to include it in any national drug provision plans.

The drug is becoming a huge success story for the UK-based pharmaceutical multinational that developed it but, as mandated by the licensing authorities, they still need to carry out post-licensure studies to update the drug safety profile by obtaining more information about rare and longer-term side-effects. With the support of a major Northern public health research agency, the pharmaceutical company decides to embark on an ambitious drug donation and evaluation programme in a West African country. The country in question is undergoing a rapid health transition characterized by an increase in chronic diseases, which is partly due to changes in smoking and dietary habits. The company and public health research agency discuss and agree their plans with leaders at the country's National Research Institute, and as a result an X-22 drug evaluation group, including international and national investigators, is established. After consultation and agreement with the Ministry of Health, the group decides to conduct the programme in a district with a population of 400,000, which has among the highest rates of coronary heart disease in the country.

The pharmaceutical company commits to donating X-22 to all of the public health facilities based within this district for three years. Patients at high risk of coronary heart disease – as determined by age, cholesterol levels, blood pressure, family history, and lifestyle habits such as smoking – are offered X-22 as part of the programme. Participation involves patients visiting their local health facility every two months for two years. At each visit, the patient's health status is checked, and they are asked to complete health and lifestyle questionnaires and provide blood samples for cholesterol monitoring. Blood tests are processed at district level and then transferred to a data server hosted by the National Research Institute, along with the other personal health information, where it is analyzed by investigators from the national and international evaluation group. To support patient care and help to process the blood samples, the pharmaceutical company funds the establishment of a small laboratory in every dispensary and a larger data-processing and laboratory facility in the district hospital.

After just one year, over 5,000 patients have consented to take part in the programme. This sparks the interest of a local journalist, who finds out how much X-22 costs and asks the pharmaceutical company what they plan to do to ensure local patients can continue to access the drug once the programme is finished. It becomes evident X-22's main target market is high-income customers, who are interested in a preventative medication to help offset high-risk behaviours such as a poor diet, smoking, and a lack of exercise. The drug has a statistically significant but relatively small effect on predicted morbidity and mortality, and is therefore not intended for populations which struggle with much more immediate, and more easily controlled, health issues. The company representative tells the local journalist that there are no immediate plans to market the drug at a lower price in his country.

In response, the journalist publishes a major article headlined 'African guinea pigs for Western lifestyle drug', arguing that the programme abuses vulnerable patients and health systems to expand the market share of a high-cost drug which will benefit only patients in very different socio-economic conditions – and, of course, the drug company. According to his article, the drug donation and evaluation programme is just a way to camouflage a for-profit drug trial. The article causes major outrage, not just among patients, but also among doctors and nurses – especially those not involved with the donation programme. One year earlier than anticipated, and in the middle of discussions about an extension of the donation programme, the pharmaceutical company decides to terminate its commitment. In a commentary in the same newspaper, the national Principal Investigator of the programme regrets the closure of the project, and comments that this could lead to significant heart problems for those taking part, which could have been avoided.

QUESTIONS

- What is your view of this programme? How would you describe it? What is the main purpose? Does it constitute research?
- Why do you think the pharmaceutical company and Northern public health agency decided to conduct the drug donation and evaluation programme in West Africa? Why is it not being conducted among those who are more likely to be able to access the drug after the study?
- What is your view of the benefits and disadvantages of making X-22 available via the programme?
- What questions would you ask to get a clearer picture of the programme and its ethical implications? You may want to think about what you would ask
    1. the different members of the drug donation and evaluation programme,
    2. national policymakers,
    3. local health facility staff,
    4. staff directing the programme at district level, and
    5. participants.
- How do you think these different stakeholders would respond? What might their views be on the relative benefits and disadvantages of the programme?
- Do you agree with the journalist? Explain why, or why not. Was it right to publish the article? What were the consequences? What did the article not achieve?
- Why did the drug company end the programme? Do you think this was right? Were there other options?
- Do you know of similar cases, in which charitable and commercial interests are mixed?

GROUP ACTIVITY

Divide into two groups, one arguing for the programme, the other against it. Think about the benefits to particular individuals at different levels of the programme, as well as large groups of people. Next, discuss and aim to agree on a list of minimum requirements that you think should be met by any drug donation programme operating in your area of work.

FURTHER READING

Pinheiro, C.P. (2008) Drug donations: what lies beneath. *Bulletin of the World Health Organization* 86(8), 580.

Saha, S. and Galper, A. (2013). The ethical basis of drug donation to third world countries. *Ethics in Biology, Engineering and Medicine* 4(1), 29–46.

Samsky, A. (2011) Since we are taking the drugs: Labor and value in two international drug donation programs. *Journal of Cultural Economy* 4(1), 27–43.

Samsky, A. (2012) Scientific sovereignty: How international drug donation programs reshape health, disease, and the state. *Cultural Anthropology* 27(2), 310–332.

Shretta, R., Walt, G., Brugha, R. and Snow, R.W. (2001) A political analysis of corporate drug donations: the example of Malarone in Kenya. *Health Policy and Planning* 16(2), 161–170.

STAFF RELATIONSHIPS

TRAINING CASE STUDIES

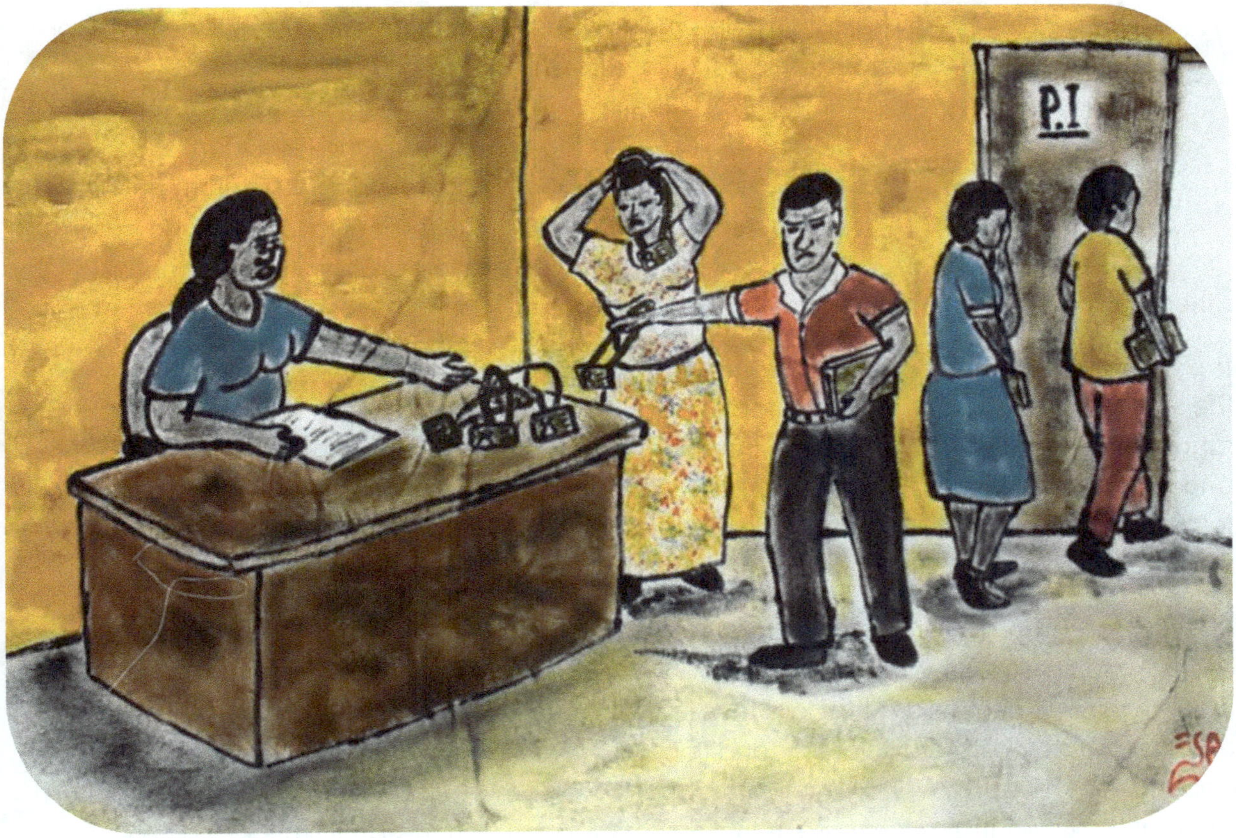

THE STAFF TURNED IN THEIR BADGES SADLY. "ANOTHER SHORT TERM CONTRACT..." THEY SIGHED.

STAFF RELATIONSHIPS

CASE STUDIES

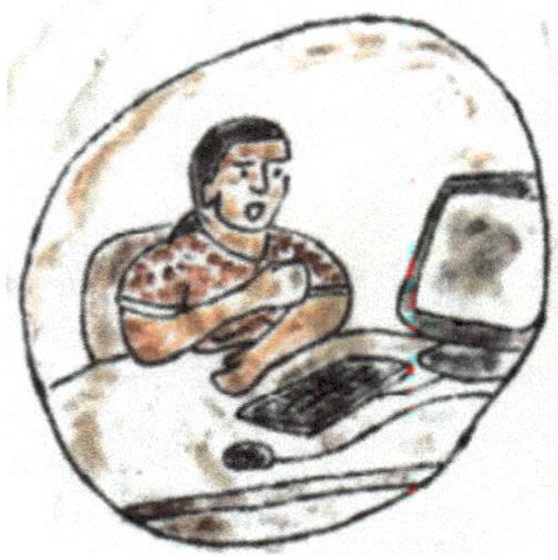

CONNECTING WITH THE WORLD

The majority of global health research in Africa is conducted through transnational organizations. These are collaborative partnerships between one or more in-country national research institutions, and the overseas arms of one or more government or academic institutions from other countries. The situation is further complicated by the involvement of global non-governmental bodies, usually through the provision of funding. Often, specific research projects are multi-sited, connecting institutions and staff in multiple sites and countries. Project-specific funding also means that whilst some staff are employed on a more permanent basis, others are employed on a contract or even daily basis.

The nature of research and its requirements means that the staff population may include people with a wide range of educational backgrounds, from highly skilled and educated scientists to community mobilizers with less formal education, chosen for their knowledge of their local communities.

FURTHER READING

Redfield P. (2012) The unbearable lightness of expats: double binds of humanitarian mobility. *Cultural Anthropology* 27(2), 358–382.

Medical research, therefore, brings together staff from different national, cultural and educational backgrounds. It also means that in one research field-station there may be groups of staff employed under different salaries, conditions and regulations – and exposed to different opportunities for educational and professional development. The stories in this section look at some of the issues that might arise in these circumstances when staff from these different backgrounds relate to one another.

Some of these stories explore the relationships between 'expatriate' researchers from the North with African researchers. The chance to experience different cultures is often a motivating factor in seeking employment in medical research on both sides. However, the differences between their socio-economic situations are difficult to avoid.

Expats are often employed on short-term contracts, their children attend international schools, and they frequently travel to international meetings and conferences. Security issues can mean they are housed in gated communities, with special guards and secure vehicles. They

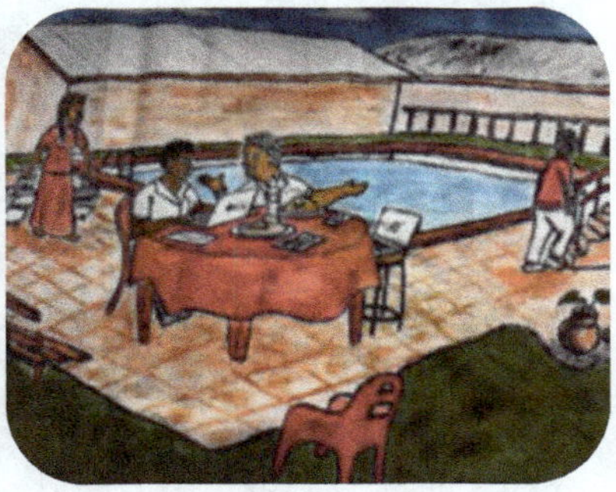

MEETING BY THE CLUB POOL

may have to follow certain rules about where they can go and what they can do whilst living in Africa. What difficulties does this pose for relationships between expat and African staff? Other stories in this section look at experiences and allegations of nepotism and corruption in medical research institutions in Africa. Perceptions – and often realities – of corruption in the public sector in Africa are high. How do these perceptions affect employment issues and staff relationships in medical research, when held by staff and communities?

PER DIEM:
PRACTICAL INEQUALITIES IN SCIENTIFIC COLLABORATION

FACILITATOR'S NOTES

This case study demonstrates how the economic circumstances of different staff shape their professional positions, and determine the practical choices they make. In this story, economic inequalities affect staff participation at a national conference. Some effects are subtle, like authorship positions, and others are more evident, like differences in accommodation and levels of physical presence at the conference. Different actors experience this situation very differently, and draw different conclusions from it.

The main aim of this case study is to think about how these inequalities emerge, sometimes in unanticipated ways; how this might affect collaboration; and how a more equitable situation could be achieved. It is important to remember that some inequalities have historical, political and economic roots, and that trying to redress the balance is not straightforward. Nonetheless it is important to engage with and discuss these inequalities in a constructive manner, to work towards lasting change. In this particular case, the discussion might lead to both simple practical changes in the way the conference is organized, and a more general consideration of long-term issues like discrepancies in salaries.

In exploring this story, students could reflect on the ways that equality is often taken for granted in professional scientific engagements. Inequality, however, persists in many ways, material and immaterial – and inequalities are perceived in various ways, filtered through different stakeholders' everyday life experience and historical memory. The ways in which we see or don't see, and engage or don't engage with, material inequalities shape how we live and work together.

LEARNING OBJECTIVE

To think about the various practical effects of inequalities between different types of staff, and to brainstorm both short-term and long-term solutions towards equality in the workplace

KEYWORDS

Employment issues

Money

North-South relationships

PER DIEM:
PRACTICAL INEQUALITIES IN SCIENTIFIC COLLABORATION

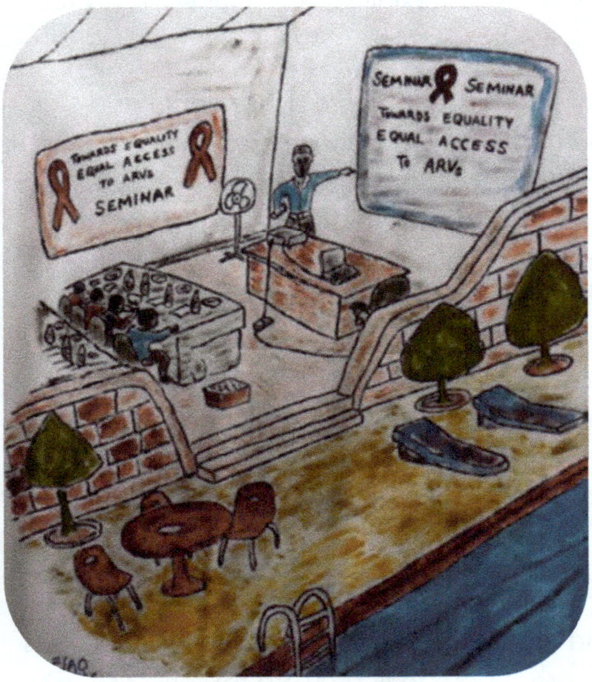

'AFTER A LONG DAY AT THE CONFERENCE, I THINK I'LL HAVE A DIP IN THE POOL...'

THE STORY

A workshop on HIV care is held in an international 4-star hotel, which offers well-equipped conference rooms, excellent catering, and pleasant garden and pool areas around which scientists can meet and talk between sessions. Rooms and meal prices are expensive, but the delegates' employers – international NGOs and their collaborators – pay a substantial per diem which covers all the costs incurred in attending the workshop, so this does not affect participation. Delegates include international policy advisors, scientists, local civil servants, and health facility personnel.

Most workshop presentations – well-prepared slide sets embossed with the relevant organizational logos – are given by African clinicians, policymakers and scientists, on behalf of co-authors who are predominantly overseas colleagues. Proceedings are carefully timed, allowing for animated and friendly discussions after each paper. The conference chairs seek to involve and elicit views from all participants, regardless of their status.

Over dinner, a leading international NGO representative states how impressed she is by the large number of African presenters at this workshop, but wonders why so few of the local healthcare staff attend dinner and evening activities. The director of a large NGO consortium which sent many staff to the conference points out that all his staff, irrespective of their nationality or seniority, receive the same per diem for their conference visit, and that it is up to individuals to decide where they stay. But, he adds, 'Maybe next time we should just pay for the hotel for everybody.'

While international visitors and most managers from larger international NGOs (local and expatriate), as well as some Northern HIV care volunteers, stay at the conference hotel, most Department of Health staff, local clinicians and civil society representatives have chosen to stay elsewhere in town, in cheaper accommodation or with relatives. Due to traffic and long commuting times, many arrive late and leave immediately after the last presentation. They receive the same per diem regardless. The same evening, some delegates including a group of local HIV activists and junior health professionals from the regional hospital have gathered at a popular music venue. Over a drink they start to discuss their respective per diem rates, and jokingly compare how much they can save from this three-day conference. Based on her US$70 per diem, one nurse calculates that she will be able to take home almost her monthly salary after tax – just at the right time, before the school fees are due. She stays with a relative, and her two hours' local transport costs less than US$2.

Two Scandinavian student volunteers tagged along on this outing, preferring the lively music venue to the hotel pool. The evening gets late, and when everybody leaves, their new friends, who are familiar with the city and its dangers, take great care to find a safe taxi driver to take them back to the hotel. The volunteers depart, slightly embarrassed, as their friends jokingly point out, 'We must take care to get you safely back home from the ghetto!'

The next morning, everybody is assembled to listen to an honorary address given by one of the host country's most eminent doctors, who is well known for his advocacy of traditional medicine. Looking at his young colleagues, he praises the progress African medicine has made since the 1960s, a time when he had to leave Africa to obtain his degree. He starts by acknowledging the achievements of the international organization hosting the conference, and then recounts his research into herbal medicines, drawing attention to the achievements of African traditional doctors. Finally, he calls for more emphasis to be placed on local resources to tackle HIV/AIDs, warning against dependency on drugs manufactured by powerful global pharmaceutical companies. After that, a young woman from the international organization which sponsored the workshop thanks the speaker, joins in his praise of African doctors, thanks the sponsors, and closes the meeting.

QUESTIONS

- Inequality appears at many different points in this account. Try to identify different forms of inequality, taking note of who is involved and how the power differences become apparent.
- Equality, as a value and intention, is also present throughout the observations presented above. Explore where and in what ways equality is emphasized.
- Why is the manager of the expatriate NGO proud of their policy regarding per diem rates? What is made equal by them (and what is not)?
- What do you think junior local doctors would say if next year their hotel bill was paid for and they received no further per diem? Would this be more equitable? Why?
- Why are the two expatriate volunteers embarrassed by their friends' joke?
- What concerns over equality and inequality are expressed in the senior doctor's honorary speech? How might this be perceived by different members of the audience?
- How does the way we engage or don't engage with material inequalities shape working relationships and research practice? Why is it difficult to talk about hidden inequalities in a situation like this? What do you think should be done?

REFLECTION ON YOUR OWN EXPERIENCES

- Which inequalities are present among staff and collaborators in your own research setting?
- Which of these inequalities are spoken about and directly addressed, and which are not?
- Are there social settings or groupings in which inequalities can be discussed, and others where one does not take them up?
- Are there practices or situations in which equality, as a moral value, is emphasized or followed through on, within your research organization?

FURTHER READING

Geissler, P. W. (2014). What future remains? Remembering an African place of science. In: Geissler, W. (ed.) *Para-states and Medical Science: Making Global Health in Africa.* Duke University Press, Durham, North Carolina, 142-178.

Redfield P. (2012) The unbearable lightness of expats: double binds of humanitarian mobility. *Cultural Anthropology* 27(2), 358–382.

Simon, C. and Mosavel, M. (2011) Getting personal: ethics and identity in global health research. *Developing World Bioethics* 11(2), 82–92.

DO ANTHROPOLOGISTS KNOW BEST?:
RELATIONSHIPS BETWEEN SOCIAL SCIENTISTS AND MEDICAL RESEARCHERS

FACILITATOR'S NOTES

This story is about misunderstandings which can occur around the role of social scientists working in collaboration with medical researchers. Through the discussion, participants will hopefully come to appreciate the anthropologist's understanding of her role as critic, and as a representative of community views. They should also understand the sensitivities of the medical scientists, who hold managerial and budgetary responsibilities as well as being concerned with the public image of their research, and try their best to do good and useful science. In particular, the story exposes different views of the concepts of validity and data in the different disciplines.

Discussing the study should leave participants with a sense of the opportunities for social science to bring difficult issues 'to the fore' and thereby respond to problems and promote improvements – but also a sense of the challenges and sensitivities which arise from practising social science in medical research.

LEARNING OBJECTIVE

To reflect on the critical role, and limitations and responsibilities, of social scientists involved in medical research

KEYWORDS

Social science

DO ANTHROPOLOGISTS KNOW BEST?:

RELATIONSHIPS BETWEEN SOCIAL SCIENTISTS AND MEDICAL RESEARCHERS

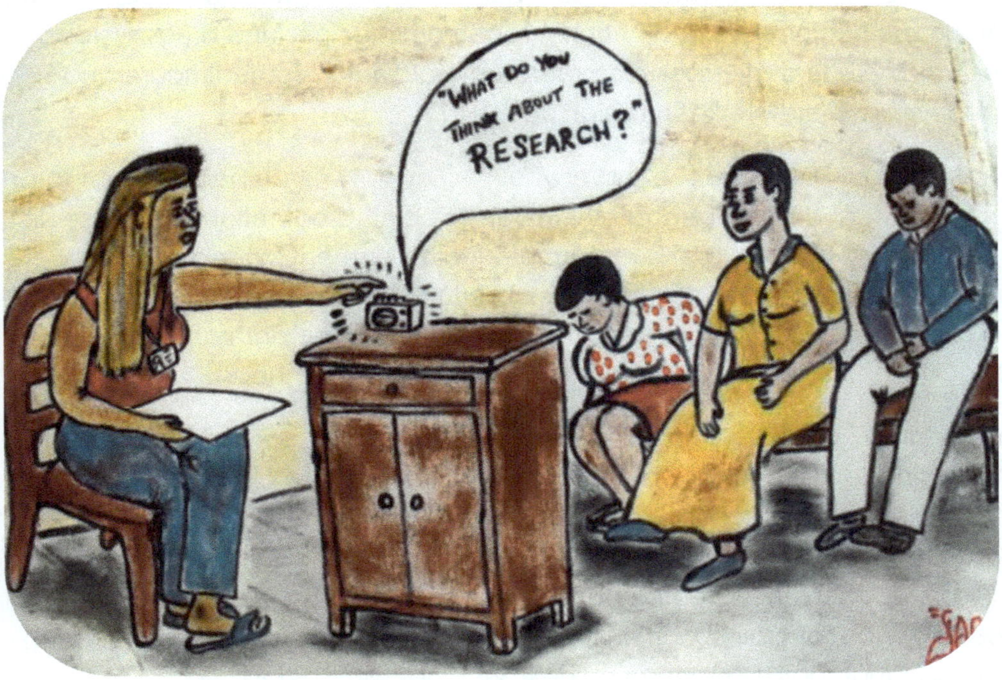

ELISE FOUND THE RESEARCH PARTICIPANTS WERE KEEN TO HAVE THEIR VOICES HEARD

THE STORY

Elise is an anthropology graduate student from a leading North American university. To bridge an employment gap before embarking on her PhD, on 'Poverty, child-death and resistance in Brazilian slums', she finds short-term employment with her university's teaching hospital, which has a long-term overseas collaborative programme conducting health research in Africa. Her task is to support a planned malaria vaccine trial, by examining how ready the community seems to be for the new study and providing social science insights. The contract also requires her to submit social science academic papers before the end of her one-year contract.

Elise sets out to conduct fieldwork among the communities from which trial participants are soon to be recruited. Working together with a local translator, she interviews people from all walks of life, and different generations and gender, about expectations and experiences of research. She expected that people would be somewhat skeptical about international research, but she very quickly learns that while former research participants and their families hold diverse views of research – some negative, most positive – they are overall extremely keen to participate in research projects.

However, people's ideas about what research is about are often far from the actual aims and practices of the studies that they have participated in. They seem to know little about which diseases actually were studied, and for what purposes blood specimens were collected. There is little awareness of the use of placebos and of unproven study vaccines and drugs; instead, the prevalent understanding is that the research programme provides top healthcare and better drugs, and people are therefore keen to sign up.

Elise finds this fascinating, partly because she is overwhelmed by how much people want to be part of research projects, and partly because her findings point to potential weaknesses in the informed consent process. It seems that a more thorough assessment is needed of how much actual information is passed on to communities about the studies. She thinks that these findings could be useful to the future trial, but also that they speak to the anthropological literature on global justice and inequality, which are subjects close to her heart.

Halfway through her fieldwork, she presents a draft manuscript at the research station's weekly seminar, entitled: '"Bring more research" – why people are so keen to join clinical trials'. In the paper, she describes the sometimes comical, sometimes worrying misunderstandings about research that she has found, and as a background she examines differences between the excellent healthcare provided by the research centre and the weaknesses of local health facilities. She argues that under overall conditions of poverty, information is ultimately less important to local people than good healthcare. She concludes with specific recommendations for improved consent procedures.

The discussion at the seminar is lively. Front-line fieldworkers, especially, confirm and expand on the misunderstandings that Elise described, underlining that, as one of them puts it, 'Participants don't really care what the research is about, as long as they get good healthcare'.

Elise's Principal Investigator is slightly critical about the paper, however, and asks: 'How representative is this?', 'How many people have you asked?', and, eventually 'So, you are saying that we completely failed to inform people about what our research is about? That their consent is essentially worthless? Have you actually done statistics on this? Do anthropologists know best?'

In a subsequent conversation between the Principal Investigator, Elise, and the overall programme director, Elise is told that the paper as it stands has scientific weaknesses and is potentially damaging to the site – also on account of the 'offensive' description of local healthcare institutions and practices. Elise, who has spent weeks writing this first paper, is sad and offended, because, as she interjects, she is supportive of global health research, and thinks these findings are important to improve the work. She convinces her Principal Investigator to allow her to rewrite the paper; eventually it is submitted, but Elise is left with the feeling that she did not say things quite as clearly as she wanted to.

QUESTIONS

- Why do you think Elise was so interested in this subject and made it her first paper?
- Why did her line managers react negatively to her material and analysis?
- What different ideas about 'data' and 'validity' might play into this discussion?
- Who do you think cares more about the wellbeing of local people, and in what ways? Does the problem lie in different disciplines, or different personal commitments?
- How would Elise have justified that her findings are relevant for medical research?

REFLECTION ON YOUR OWN EXPERIENCES

- In what way do you think anthropology could make a useful contribution to health research?
- What do anthropologists have to look out for when writing about such issues?
- What is required from medical scientists to allow for fruitful collaboration with social scientists?

FURTHER READING

Lederman, R. (2007) Comparative "research": A modest proposal concerning the object of ethics regulation. *PoLAR: Political and Legal Anthropology Review* 30(2): 305-327.

Bell, K. and Elliott, D. (2014) Censorship in the name of ethics: critical public health research in the age of human subjects regulation. *Critical Public Health* 24(4): 385-391.

WHO ARE YOU?:
EMPLOYMENT ISSUES AND NORTH-SOUTH RELATIONSHIPS

FACILITATOR'S NOTES

This case study is about the relationship between local scientific staff and expatriates, and the experiences and perceptions of employment status which might affect these relations. Specifically, it tells the story of a Northern PhD student who temporarily works as a well-paid consultant, and the way in which this negatively affects his previously good relations with local colleagues and advisors. In a post-colonial context of transnational medical research, staff at local host institutions and expatriates are often employed on different terms and through different mechanisms – often holding contracts with different institutions in different places.

The story invites us to think about an issue which can be very sensitive for everyone involved – who gets jobs and why in transnational medical research. And the most difficult question – what role does a person's skin colour or country of origin play in this? Following on from the central tenet of this workbook – that we believe it is important to talk about concerns that might otherwise remain unvoiced – the facilitator should use this case study as a chance to address these sensitive issues.

The first key relationship to explore here is between the PhD student and the fieldwork supervisor, which changes when the student turns into a well-paid consultant. You can imagine the fieldwork supervisor thinking, 'How did this happen? How did he gain the ear of the European director so quickly? Why was I not given the same opportunity?' His subsequent refusal to engage with the project could be read as a way to regain some power in the situation. The story then becomes a lesson in how to properly handle employment issues, in order to render decisions transparent.

LEARNING OBJECTIVE

To reflect upon unspoken assumptions and challenges in relation to personal economic circumstances and professional roles, when Northern scientists and students work in Southern medical research sites

KEYWORDS

Employment issues

North-South relationships

Capacity building

WHO ARE YOU?:
EMPLOYMENT ISSUES AND NORTH-SOUTH RELATIONSHIPS

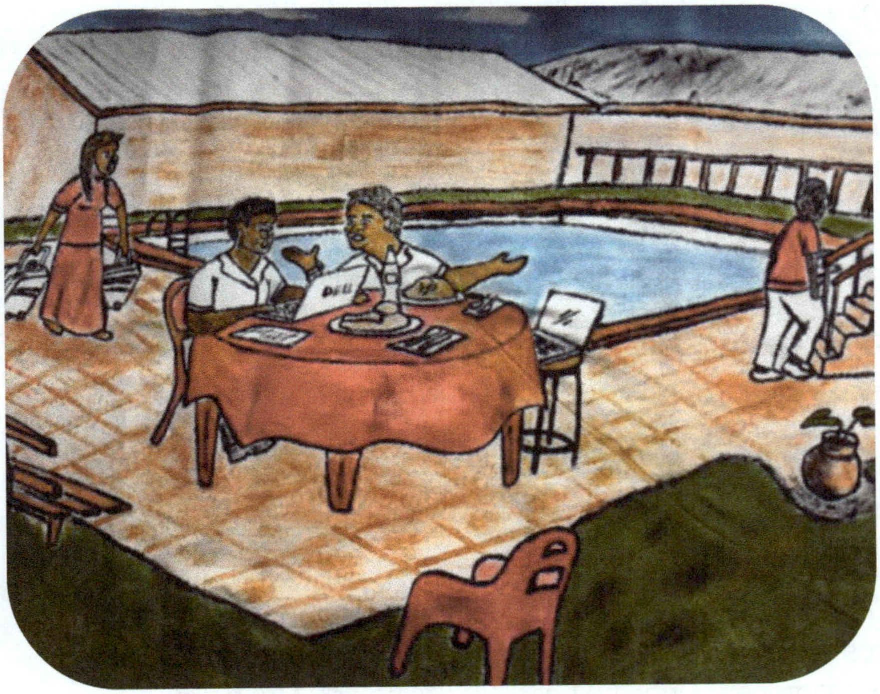

MOHAMMED SAW ANTONIS THE PI TALKING TO JAMES AT THE CLUB....

THE STORY

James is a 35-year-old German PhD student at Hamburg University, with a background in computer science and developing digital health technologies for projects in Germany and overseas. In his PhD he wants to assess how electronic systems and digital devices are being used to collect demographic and health-related data at household level, and help develop more sophisticated and user-friendly systems for use in resource-limited settings. One of James' PhD supervisors has international contacts with a Tanzanian research station, which is mainly funded by the European and Developing Countries Clinical Trials Partnership (EDCTP). He puts James in contact with the directors and they agree that he can come for a preliminary visit to explore the feasibility of conducting his research at the station.

During his visit James is shown around the research facilities, and introduced to Tanzanian members of staff who work in the IT and demographic surveillance offices. They are welcoming and the demographic surveillance fieldwork supervisor, Mohammed, who is completing a Masters in health informatics, is particularly interested in James' ideas. James decides to include him as a co-investigator on his protocol.

During his visit, James also meets Antonis, the European Senior Scientist, who is responsible for the conduct of research funded by EDCTP. They meet formally at the station to discuss James' proposed PhD project and also socially for dinner at one of the restaurants frequented by expatriates in the city. Antonis knows that James has a background in computer science and digital health and so asks him to help draw up the job description for an e-health research coordinator. He also asks James if he knows anyone from his past work who would be willing to apply for the position as a short-term consultancy, with a view to training a Tanzanian researcher to take it over.

On his return to Hamburg James prepares his research protocol for ethics review. His new Tanzanian collaborators tell him that obtaining Tanzanian ethics clearance will take a long time and is easier to work on in-country. James is keen to get started on things in Tanzania as his PhD funding is time-limited. So he decides to apply for the e-health research coordinator position himself. The consultancy fees will augment his research funds, cover his living expenses and enable him to move to Tanzania earlier. James is invited for interview and returns to Tanzania where he is interviewed by four national and international researchers based at the medical research station.

James is offered the job and starts to juggle pushing through the national and European ethics clearance for his PhD research, with mentoring a Tanzanian IT graduate and working closely with other IT staff and health researchers. Once he has settled in he asks Mohammed, the demographic surveillance fieldwork supervisor, if he could spend some time with him in the field observing how fieldworkers collect data. Mohammed responds negatively and advises his team not to let him join them in any fieldwork activities. James is baffled – and a little hurt – and does not know what to do. Mohammed had initially seemed so supportive of his PhD plans. Now, his resistance to James' work could be very detrimental to both his PhD fieldwork and his good relations with his new colleagues.

QUESTIONS

- Why does James decide to take up the consultancy work? Why is he offered it?
- Consider how this work might affect his PhD research both positively and negatively.
- Why does Mohammed's attitude towards James' PhD research change?
- What should James do?

REFLECTION ON YOUR OWN EXPERIENCES

- Have you ever witnessed or been in a similar situation? Who do you identify with in this story and why?
- What processes could be put in place to mitigate potential tensions as a result of James's employment?

FURTHER READING

Redfield P. (2012) The unbearable lightness of expats: double binds of humanitarian mobility. *Cultural Anthropology* 27(2), 358–382.

Okwaro, F.M. and Geissler, P.W. (2015). In/dependent Collaborations: Perceptions and experiences of African scientists in transnational HIV research. *Medical Anthropology Quarterly* http://dx.doi.org/10.1111/maq.12206

Prince, R.J. (2013) "Tarmacking" in the millennium city: spatial and temporal trajectories of empowerment and development in Kisumu, Kenya. *Africa: Journal of the International African Institute* 83, 582–605.

Nordling, L. (2014) Kenyan doctors win landmark discrimination case, *Nature* 22 July 2014

Irikefe, V. et al (2011) Science in Africa: The view from the front line. Published online 29 June 2011, *Nature* 474, 556-559 doi:10.1038/474556a.

SNOT FOR SALE:
STAFF'S HANDLING OF TRANSPORT REIMBURSEMENT AND RUMOURS

FACILITATOR'S NOTES

The main aim of this story is to encourage reflection on the way rumours arise and are dealt with in a medical research setting. It focuses particularly on the role of money in rumours, as well as how junior staff deal with such rumours and why, sometimes, they may not feel comfortable discussing their experiences with senior colleagues. It concerns a rumour, heard by village health workers working on the study, that researchers are buying and reselling children's snot.

There is often a great deal of concern in the medical research world about rumours which associate research in Africa with blood stealing, Satanism and witchcraft. Narratives about blood stealing are found all over sub-Saharan Africa; blood has both literal and metaphorical power in many settings and most research stations will be implicated in such rumours at some point. This story deals with a more mundane bodily substance for rumour: snot. This also allows the training group to focus on the fact that the cause of rumours is related not only to what medical researchers do in medical procedural terms (like taking blood), but also what they are doing in social and economic terms.

This story is useful for thinking about the practice of providing transport reimbursement in medical research, and how something seemingly straightforward may prove complex in practice. Some of the mothers whose children are participating in the study perceive their transport reimbursement as payment for services or products rendered. Are they right? How does this practice feature in and contribute to the rumour? This story shows how certain 'micro' issues, such as the specific study procedures for disseminating results, and the timing of the distribution of money allocated

LEARNING OBJECTIVE

To reflect on the role of money in rumours about medical research, and the challenges facing field staff around dealing with rumours and discussing them with senior colleagues

KEYWORDS

Money

Employment issues

Rumour

Informed consent

Inducements

for transport reimbursements, contribute to the rumour. But you might also want to think about the role of 'macro' issues or relations, such as historical social and economic relationships between the West African country and the countries of its research collaborators.

Whilst rumours can sometimes be very damaging to medical research activities, it is important to remember that rumours are not fixed ideas. They are unstable, open-ended, and often debated and reframed in face-to-face contact. In this story the rumour ultimately did not affect research participation. Invite your group to think about why this might be so.

Rumours can teach us about the dynamics of social relationships. Both the rumour itself and the way it is discussed amongst the medical researchers can tell us something about the social relationships operating here – not only between the villagers and the researchers, but also between the study coordinator and the village health workers. The village reporters described below do not feel able to raise the issue of the rumour with the study coordinator. They keep quiet. Encourage the group to discuss why. This story can also be used, therefore, to enable staff to 'deliberate' how best to encourage junior and senior colleagues to engage in open discussion about challenges and understandings of study procedures.

SNOT FOR SALE:
STAFF'S HANDLING OF TRANSPORT REIMBURSEMENT AND RUMOURS

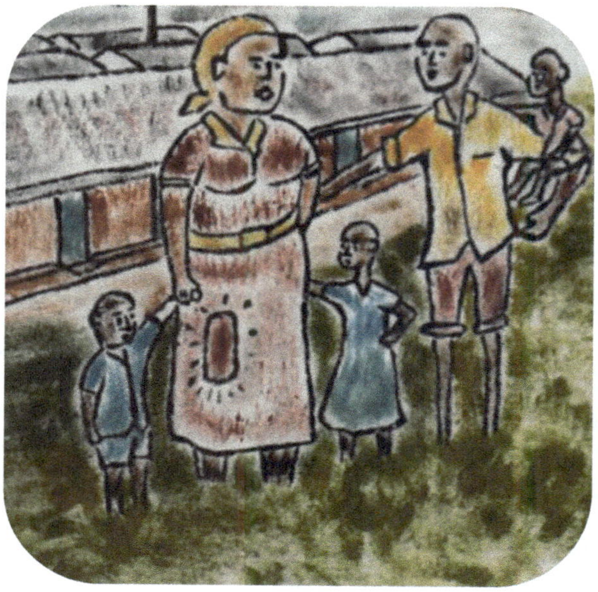

"DID YOU HEAR? THOSE STRANGE RESEARCHERS ARE BUYING CHILDREN'S SNOT!"

THE STORY

In some villages in a West African country, mothers are asked to bring their children to a clinic so researchers can collect nasal swab samples to check for certain viruses. Each village has its own village health worker who is employed by the transnational research station. The village health workers are respected locally, know the people well, and act as a link between the villagers and the researchers. The study pays them to invite the mothers to come to the clinic. They walk door to door visiting the mothers and telling them about the study. Each mother who decides to takes her child is told she will be given a small sum of money to cover her transport costs. She is also told that she won't be given her child's individual results because they will not be able to tell if the presence of the viruses mean the child is sick. But at the end of the study the researchers will give a presentation about the overall findings.

Halfway through recruitment, the study coordinator calls a meeting with the village health workers. A similar study was conducted in this area last year, but so far, the number of children recruited is lower this year, despite the researchers being able to offer more transport reimbursement. The study coordinator wants to know why. He asks the village health workers for their opinions. The village health workers are non-committal. It has been raining a lot lately so perhaps the mothers are too busy farming, they offer. Or perhaps it is because the swabbing hurts the children? Another suggests that increasing the transport reimbursement might help. The study coordinator tells the village health workers that increasing the reimbursements is impossible. 'We have to give everybody the same amounts,' he tells them, 'and some of your participants are able to walk to the clinic anyway.'

A social scientist, Joe, who has been working and living in the village, is also at the meeting. He has heard a rumour that some mothers don't want to take part, because they suspect that if researchers are prepared to buy something strange like snot, there must be a sinister reason. Perhaps, they wonder, it is what Americans use in witchcraft instead of blood.

'*Buy* the snot?' Joe says to the mothers when he hears this. 'What makes you think they are *buying* it?' The mothers explain that after the samples are taken from their children, they are given some money. To them this was a clear commercial transaction. 'Isn't that money for your transport?' Joe asks. 'How could it be?' the mothers reply. 'Most of us live within walking distance to the clinic, and anyway we are given the money afterwards, not before.'

'Also,' one of the mothers says, 'a friend of mine who lives a bit far did ask the researchers to pay the motorbike driver who carried her to the clinic. They refused. They told her she had to wait to get her payment until the sample was taken. And the driver was waiting right there for the money. He charged her waiting fees!'

Joe wonders if he should say anything in the meeting about this rumour. In the break he asks some of the village health workers if they have heard it too. 'Oh yes,' they reply, 'everyone is talking about it, and part of the problem is that it is very hard to explain to the mothers why they don't get their child's individual results. To be honest, we don't really understand either.'

Joe asks them how they explain the transport reimbursement to those mothers who live within walking distance of the clinic. Anna, a village health worker famous for her sense of humour, tells him, 'Oh, I say, "You know, you could take a motorbike to the clinic. Or you could walk like this and this [miming a winding route with her hand] and cut through your neighbour's compound like *this*, and through the market like *this*, where you buy some refreshing soda to keep you going!"'

Joe tells them it might be helpful for the study coordinator to know about the rumour and the challenges. He asks the village health workers to bring it up after the break. But they don't. At the end of the meeting Joe raises his hand and tells the study coordinator about the rumour.

The study coordinator asks the village health workers if they have heard it. The room is quiet. Eventually, one of the health workers says they have heard the rumour, but it is just coming from one or two people; they have explained the study to them and now they are satisfied. The study coordinator sternly tells the group that the research station does *not* buy and sell samples. The matter is considered dealt with and the meeting ends.

Joe feels a little bit embarrassed and annoyed with the village health workers. 'Hey,' he says, 'why didn't you back me up in the meeting?' 'Well,' they tell him, 'researchers don't like to hear about rumours. It's our job to explain the study properly to the mothers.'

Recruitment for the study continues. The rumours also continue but don't seem to have a significant effect on the study. By the end of the study the numbers recruited are sufficient and the researchers are pleased.

QUESTIONS

- Were the researchers buying the snot?
- What might be the reasons behind the rumours? Do these have any relationship to 'reality'? You may want to think about specific local issues, and also wider historical issues.
- What does the situation tell you about how well the researchers seem to understand the local environment?
- Why do you think the village health workers were reluctant to discuss the rumours with the study coordinator? Would it have been helpful for him to know about them? What do you think he might say?
- The issue of how to administer transport reimbursement is often tricky. Are there any different ways it could have been organized here? What are the pros and cons of these ways?
- What else do you think the researchers could have done differently here to help the study run more smoothly?
- Why do you think the rumour didn't seem to have a negative effect on the study outcomes?

REFLECTIONS ON YOUR OWN EXPERIENCE

Have you experienced a particular rumour in your medical research? What conclusions can you come to if you try to 'read' it as a message to be translated? What can it tell you about social relationships? What were the specific local and wider issues contributing to it?

FURTHER READING

Fairhead, J., Leach, M., and Small, M. (2006) Where techno-science meets poverty: medical research and the economy of blood in The Gambia, West Africa. *Social Science and Medicine*, 63(4), 1109–1120.

Geissler, P.W. (2005) 'Kachinja are coming!': encounters around medical research work in a Kenyan village. *Africa: Journal of the International African Institute* 75, 173–202.

Geissler, W. (2011b) 'Transport to where?': reflections on the problem of value and time *à propos* an awkward practice in medical research. *Journal of Cultural Economy* 4(1), 45–64.

Geissler, P.W. and Pool, R. (2006) Editorial: Popular concerns about medical research projects in sub-Saharan Africa – a critical voice in debates about medical research ethics. *Tropical Medicine & International Health* 11(7), 975–982. Available at: http://onlinelibrary.wiley.com/doi/10.1111/j.1365-3156.2006.01682.x/pdf (accessed 25 October 2015.)

Kelly, A.H. and Wenzel Geissler, P. (2011) Introduction: The value of transnational medical research. *Journal of Cultural Economy* 4(1), 3–10.

Kingori, P. et al. (2010) 'Rumours' and clinical trials: a retrospective examination of a paediatric malnutrition study in Zambia, southern Africa. *BMC Public Health* 10(1), 556.

I'M SURE YOU'LL GIVE HER A CHANCE: EMPLOYMENT AND CORRUPTION

FACILITATOR'S NOTES

Transnational medical research organizations, operating in countries with limited employment opportunities, are often perceived as highly desirable places to work. Competition for employment is usually fierce. In addition, such research is heavily dependent on maintaining the goodwill of key stakeholders and target communities. In this story, one of the local government officials pressurizes a study coordinator to employ a family member. It is often difficult for research coordinators to know how to respond to this kind of situation.

It may be difficult to encourage staff to open up about this topic in a group discussion. Care should be taken to set up ground rules. For example, you might choose to ask participants to talk only about 'hypothetical' cases when reflecting on their own experiences, or examples from other organizations they have worked with. If you aim to use this case study to support your human resources policy, it would be important to have this to hand, and to encourage participants to talk about possible challenges they may face in following these rules.

LEARNING OBJECTIVE

To acknowledge the difficult issue of corruption in the employment processes of medical research organizations, and to discuss how to address this

KEYWORDS

Money

Employment issues

Corruption

Government

I'M SURE YOU'LL GIVE HER A CHANCE:
EMPLOYMENT AND CORRUPTION

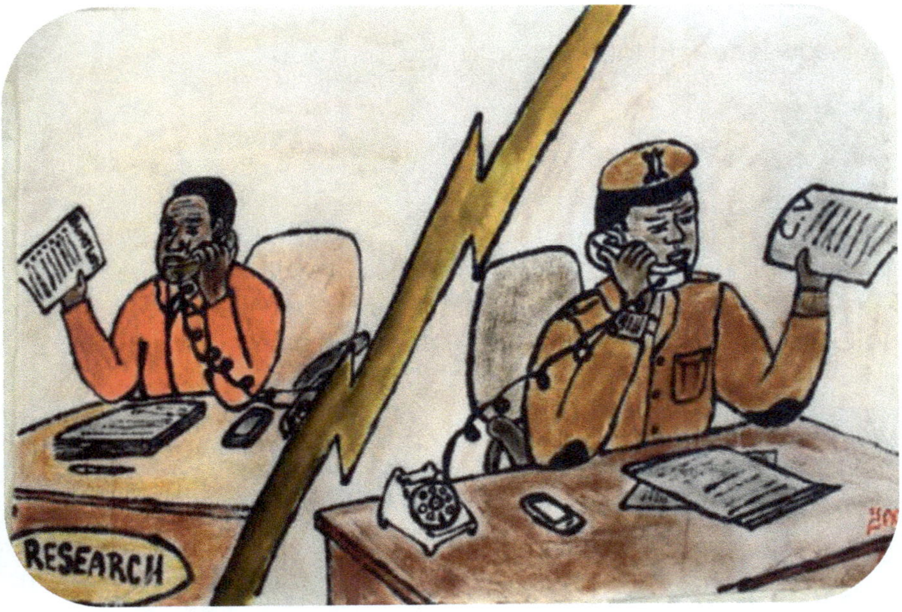

DAVID JUST COULD NOT GET THE CHIEF OFF THE PHONE. 'FINE,' HE SAID EVENTUALLY, 'I'LL GIVE HER A CHANCE.'

THE STORY

David is the on-site Principal Investigator for a study looking at diarrheal disease in Southern Africa. The overseas Principal Investigators have entrusted him with employing staff for the study, and ensuring smooth relations with the local administration, which is particularly important as the study involves working with primary schools. The first step is to get the local government administrators on board, as people in this region will look to them for permission to participate in any research.

The first local government meeting goes well, but after the meeting David gets a phone call from one of the officials. The official, Willis, tells him that he has a sister-in-law who would like to work on the project. David tells Willis that the application process is open to all qualified candidates, and if she has the relevant certificates she is welcome to apply. Willis replies that he is 'sure my sister-in-law will get a chance'.

When the applications come into Human Resources, Willis' sister-in-law is not shortlisted. She doesn't have the required certificates. David receives another phone call from Willis. He is very angry that the research study has 'failed to give her a chance'. He threatens to withdraw his support for the study. Panicking, David suggests that Willis' sister-in-law should apply for the next round of jobs, which have less stringent requirements. This time the sister-in-law is successful. However, Willis calls again to complain, this time about the salary which is lower than the previous position. Again he threatens to withdraw his support. David doesn't know what to do. In the end, he agrees to appoint her as a 'team leader' in her job category, and adjusts the salary a little.

A few weeks later Willis' sister-in-law is caught falsifying data and dismissed.

QUESTIONS

- What do you think will happen next?
- What beliefs lie behind the opinion that all applicants must be treated 'equally'?
- Can you see the situation from Willis' point of view? What beliefs might lie behind his behaviour?
- Do you think David was right to do what he did? What could he have done differently?
- Do you think the study would have suffered if David had not employed Willis' sister-in-law?

REFLECTIONS ON YOUR OWN EXPERIENCES

- Do you think such situations are a common occurrence in your organization?
- Can you identify similar situations, where people may be hired for reasons other than their specific skills? What reasons can you think of?
- What do you think the long-term consequences of employment practices like these might be?

ACTIVITY

Look together at your organization's hiring policy. Can you make any suggestions about how it could be improved?

GUIDANCE FOR FACILITATORS

This resource has been designed as a flexible tool for training and development. The collection of training case studies can be used by individuals or in groups.

INDIVIDUAL USE

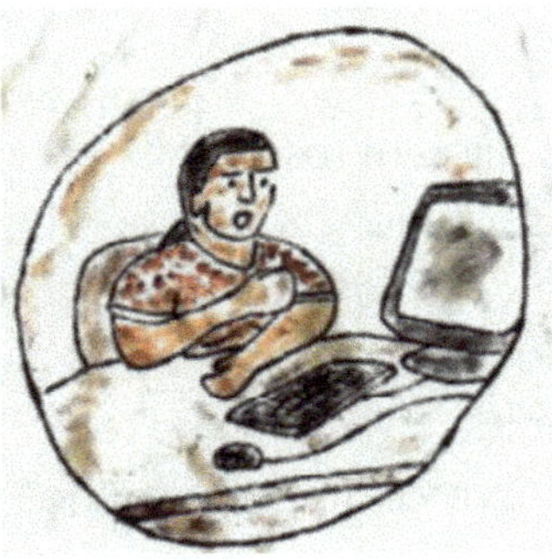

Individual readers might find it useful to read through the entire collection, or to pick stories at random, in order to draw parallels to their own experience and reflect on these. As such, this book can be read like any other. Recommended journal articles on the main themes (keywords) of each case study are provided for further reading.

GROUP USE

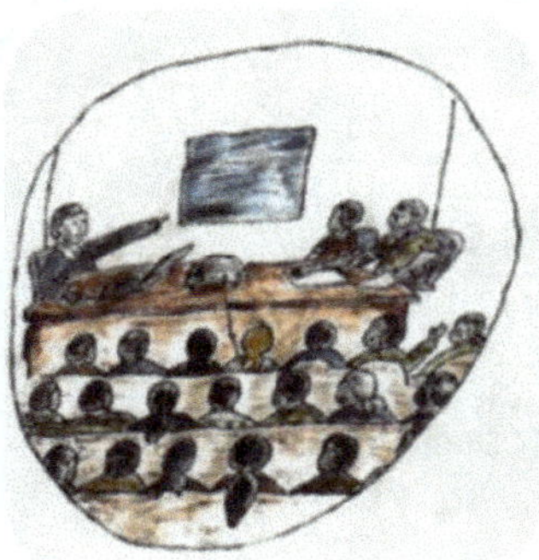

However, the workbook is mainly directed at groups of people involved in transnational medical research – either in research sites, or in academic institutions and universities – who can use the cases to elicit group discussions. This could happen during a dedicated training event, such as an ethics workshop or seminar over one or more days, involving a professional group or interested staff. If this involves many participants, smaller groups could work through single cases and report their experiences back to the larger group. Gradually, the group would in this way acquire deliberation skills and identify key issues that are of concern to them. We provide more practical information for facilitators below.

Given the pressure on time, and the difficulty of gathering staff for longer periods of time, a more efficient way of using this material might be to have short, but regular, sessions of 15 to 60 minutes to discuss one case at a time in relevant local groups. Such sessions can be added to existing meetings. For example, the members of an ethics review board, or an institutional scientific committee, could pick and discuss one case for 20 minutes before or after their monthly meetings. Here, one group member could introduce each case, and/or prepare questions and guide the debate. Similarly, a group of fieldworkers, or a Community Advisory

Board might use a relevant case to start off their regular meetings, in order to help people to think jointly through issues they confront in their daily work.

CHOICE OF TRAINING MATERIALS

In some cases, virtually any of the case stories might be relevant for a particular group (for example, scientists who as Principal Investigators bridge between academia and the field). In other cases the table of contents, keywords and summaries will help to identify particularly interesting or relevant cases relative to a particular site, target group or issue.

TRAINING GROUND RULES

In any of these cases of group deliberation, facilitators who engender sufficient respect and authority are needed to guide the discussion and encourage openness. At the same time, it is important that facilitators are not direct line managers, who might be seen as evaluating participants' responses. For example, at collaborative research sites, the local social scientist might be a good facilitator. Or, members of a group of peers might decide to rotate the role of facilitator, giving each of them an opportunity to develop their skills. Overall, it is crucial that all participants are aware that the cases are not meant to lead to definite 'correct' answers, but to create a space to voice doubts, and to admit lack of clarity and even antagonism. The aim of deliberation is to elicit different opinions and to negotiate these. Moreover, ethical deliberation has the potential to open dormant controversies among staff – indeed, this could be seen as one of its purposes. But this needs to be carefully managed to avoid negative effects on collaboration and morale (see below).

If the facilitator decides to suggest ground rules, such as confidentiality around any experiences or views discussed, it is important to ensure that all members of the group fully agree to these, and understand why an open discussion is important. The difference between apparent compliance and real commitment may be subtle, but the consequences for individual staff members might be severe.

FACILITATOR'S ROLE AND PREPARATION

The facilitator of ethical deliberation sessions, and to a certain extent the training attendees and their managers, are responsible for ensuring that discussions are underpinned by mutual respect even where differences in option emerge. Facilitators also need to manage the deliberation carefully so that the process leads to greater openness and to agreement, rather than to entrenched conflicts and disagreements.

We have provided some guidance for facilitators at the start of each case study to support constructive deliberation. However, the strength of this approach, and of the stories that we have selected, is that each of them elicits a variety of concerns and can lead to very different discussions in interaction with particular participants, or in the context of specific situations. Therefore, we cannot – and do not want – to provide exhaustive guidance. Instead, it is crucial that the facilitator thoroughly prepares for her/his task. Below, we provide some generic guidance for this.

In the most practical terms, we envisage that deliberation sessions would consist of a brief introduction by the facilitator, perhaps explaining any 'ground rules' or the fact that no 'easy answers' are to be expected. This would be followed by a period of individual reading (or reading out loud) to familiarize participants with the case. The facilitator would then encourage the participants to address the guiding questions in turn. To make it easier for participants to talk, the facilitator might ask some open questions like, 'What is happening here?' or 'What are the key ethical issues at stake here?' Later on, they could try to help participants draw upon their own experiences in relation to the case: 'Has anyone experienced similar situations?' This may, however, just arise naturally in the course of discussions.

The conversation might diverge far from the original questions; this is desirable, if it brings out local moral debates and applications. The discussion is likely to generate local comparisons and related anecdotes. Such concrete examples will enhance the discussion, but facilitators need to be mindful of the potential of underlying disagreements and conflicts to erupt (such as between field staff and scientists), which may need to be mediated. This moderation will require some skill from the facilitator, so it may be advisable to begin working with this book by starting with more general and less contentious issues.

Some advance consideration of the following questions is essential:

What is the learning objective?

When preparing for her/his task, the facilitator should first stipulate specific 'learning objectives', bearing in mind the needs of the institution, the task at hand, and the specific group selected for training. What questions should be raised, and what insights be gained? What is it reasonable to expect as an outcome to the debate? It may also be important to manage the expectations of other, senior colleagues in this regard.

What are the potential risks of using this story?

The facilitator must also think carefully about the 'risks' involved in discussing a particular story: is this the right audience, the right time, the right place for this debate? Can the target audience understand the ethical or technical dimensions of this case? Could the discussion exacerbate existing tensions, either between members of the target group, or between the group and others (managers, participants)?

What is the best training method for my group?

Once the learning objectives have been formulated and case stories chosen, taking potential risks into account, the facilitator must decide on suitable methods. Should the story be told or read? Should it be distributed during the session, or emailed beforehand? Should illustrations be used? Does the group invite smaller group work, or plenary discussion? How should smaller groups be composed, and what feedback asked for? Should one draw parallels with ongoing discussions on site, or not?

What directions might the discussion take?

Then, the facilitator should go through the case on their own, identifying the various multiple directions the discussion might take. From this, possible secondary learning aims can be derived, as well as, importantly, identifying 'dead ends' and 'detrimental controversies' to avoid. If possible, understanding something about the background of ethical dilemmas your participants have faced will be very important in this.

Our goal is for ethical deliberations on these case studies to touch on three distinct arenas of debate and action: debate over individual choices and behaviour, debate over institutional practices, and debate over wider 'structural' issues. An awareness of all three of these 'levels' operating in global medical research is, in our view, essential for participants to move forward with a wider and more empowered understanding of ethical dilemmas. See the example of the discussion of the case of 'Helping hand' below for an example of these three ethical arenas.

What is my desired outcome of the training?

Finally, it is helpful to imagine the desired endpoint of the discussion, and to prepare a 'destination' which can help the facilitator to draw together the discussion and reflect the learning aims. The facilitator might plan for this point of arrival to be reached via 1-3 points covered in the discussion, which they will want to reiterate in conclusion. Even though this 'endpoint' may contain diverse or divergent ethical views, these should be 'held' and acknowledged by all in the final summing-up, rather than participants departing in major disagreement.

All this will inevitably imply some didactic imposition on the part of the facilitator, but it avoids participants' leaving the session feeling frustrated. Good skills in facilitation are important at every point in discussing the cases, but especially in the ending of the sessions. On the one hand there is a risk that participants will leave with an overwhelming sense of futility: 'We have talked and talked, but what can be done?' Or, 'The underlying issues are so big that we can't really do anything'. On the other, they might depart with a sense of too much certainty, be it about the perceived right course of action, or, worse, about already doing things right: 'This would never have happened to us.' 'That nurse was really useless.' 'What was that PI thinking of?'

Once again it is important to reiterate that, when carefully balanced, ethical deliberation should lead to greater awareness of underlying fundamental challenges – and the impossibility of doing away with or avoiding them – *combined with* some ideas about key areas of practice where improvements are possible.

EXAMPLE: 'HELPING HAND'

Imagine you are preparing a session drawing on the case story **Helping hand.** Let us say the target group are locally trained nurses and doctors who have been employed by the research organization for between one and ten years, and work on clinical trials which recruit participants from public health facilities, and refer them for in-patient care. The seminar is originally planned for up to 20 participants.

The overall learning aim is: 'For participants to achieve a greater awareness of the diversity of viewpoints and interests, and potential for friction – among healthcare personnel, research staff and patients – involved in collaborations between government medical facilities and transnational medical research collaborations'. This could further be split up into specific aims related to: mutual perception of professional status and role (how people see each other); styles of communication (culture, gender and generation); diverging ethics of patient care, data collection and cooperation (potentially different priorities); reflection on material differences and resource use (e.g. what drugs and technologies are available or not available, and what can be done about it); etc.

Once some learning aims have been chosen, taking into account the current needs of the target population and institution, the facilitator might reflect in advance on the risks of discussing the case. Have there been any events in the recent past which might make individual participants feel uncomfortable with this discussion – e.g. conflicts between supervisors and staff, or between research staff and care staff – or which could open up undesirable conflicts among participants?

Along with the risks, you might consider the potential advantages of extending the group beyond its original constituency – for example, including local health facility staff among the deliberation participants. How would you make use of this opportunity to involve more people? How would you mitigate potential risks of doing so? Let's assume that on this occasion, you go back and invite personnel from the local health facilities, increasing the seminar size to 30+.

Then, you would design methods and an overall schedule. First, a suitable introduction needs to be sketched: Why should we discuss this topic? What are our experiences in this area? What is our overall aim (formulating this positively and inclusively, e.g. in terms of good collaboration of mutual benefit)? You decide that following the brief introduction, the participants, whom you decide will be happy with written information, will be given the case story, and suitable time to read. Given the size of the seminar group, it will then be split up into five groups of six people to discuss the case. Each group will choose a representative who will feed back to the plenary, before opening up the general discussion. You might decide that, in order to facilitate mutual understanding, the smaller groups will mix research staff and healthcare personnel.

Before the actual session, you would go through the case story carefully and identify potential directions which the discussion might take, as well as different levels of deliberation. You might write these down, as leading questions which you can raise later to help you to guide the discussion if needed. Thus, you might expect the discussion to focus on the actors' individual behaviour: Why did the research nurse behave the way she did? Could she not have done X? How is her behaviour perceived by the matron? Was his supervisor reacting correctly? How could the research nurse and the supervisor have dealt with the situation differently? Why don't the healthcare personnel do their job properly? Is the research nurse not obliged to produce good data? What interest does the local nurse have in data production? These questions point to learning aims on the level of individual behaviour and communication, enhancing awareness about the role of language, specific actions, and interactions.

One could also imagine that the discussion might turn to institutional practices: how was the research project introduced to healthcare personnel? What sort of agreement exists between the research and the healthcare institution? Is this in writing and accessible to staff? Does it specify particular practices and resources? How often do representatives and staff from the institutions formally meet, and at which level? What ownership in research results (and publications) is there on the health facility side? Are doctors included among authors, or have access to academic training? What sorts of stereotypes exist with regard to the other group?

These types of questions point to learning aims on an intermediary level, pertaining to institutional practices and structures. Awareness of these constraints and possibilities is equally important as awareness of the role of personal behaviours and choices. But it is also important that the facilitator helps the participants to think of the two areas as *distinct arenas* of reflection and action.

Questions and debates relative to these individual and institutional levels of the case story can be guided towards improved practice. You might anticipate that your group might decide that research nurses working within public healthcare institutions need adequate training about formal procedures and communication; they also need procedures, if necessary, to complain about practices which negatively affect data collection. Transnational research organizations implementing clinical trials in public hospitals, on the other hand, might need to respect the 'ownership' of local healthcare personnel, and institutionalize regular exchanges, as well as material support. While it does not serve the purpose of the deliberation seminar to identify definite solutions, it is possible here to collect propositions towards best practice, and even to ask whether any particular measures should be taken in the particular site.

Finally, it is hoped that the discussion will not only touch on these arenas of personal and institutional arrangements, but also reach a different level altogether: that of 'structural' political-economic relations of inequality. How can a research organization improve healthcare, if the state is unable to do so? Isn't this a bottomless pit? Must the research organization not protect its resources, in order to produce good data? Or: Why has the research organization worked in this hospital for two decades, without significantly improving hospital practices? Shouldn't transnational researchers contribute to local healthcare, or train local doctors? But also: Isn't good data an important contribution to improved local healthcare? If not, why do scientific research findings not always translate into local healthcare benefits?

These questions point towards global inequalities at the global level. As such, it is much more difficult to find clear-cut ways forward. You can expect some participants to propose unequivocal 'solutions': the mandate of research organizations is only to do research; besides, they should not alter local healthcare realities, because this would affect the validity and local relevance of their findings. Moreover, it would be unethical to improve healthcare and thus induce patients and hospitals to agree to research. Other participants might argue the opposite: to act ethically, large international research organizations should significantly improve or even build the hospitals they research in. Here, the facilitator's skill is required to steer away from a polarization, and to avoid simple solutions. On this 'macro' of deliberation, rather, the learning aim should be to recognise the inevitable fact that transnational medical research is situated within what may be termed 'structural violence' related to the distribution of power and resources, and this has a direct effect on human lives.

Thinking about how this plays out in any given situation will, hopefully, not simply raise but also help to answer the question of 'what's the point?' Touching on this area is challenging, but it can also be energizing; it provides the underlying motivation of many thousands of people from all backgrounds working in global medical research around the world. A logical end point of your group's deliberation process might be that they decide both individuals and institutions have an ongoing and continuous responsibility to work for improvements, to strive to 'make things better', without being able to resolve the underlying contradictions. In this sense, the authors of this workbook believe that the overall take-home message of discussing these cases could be formulated as: 'we can all do more, and we must keep trying'. This, then, would be the 'destination' to be aimed for by the facilitator. A case like 'Helping hand' raises ethical concerns pertaining to three major levels: individual, institutional, and global-structural. While the first two arenas provide opportunities to do things a little better – improving patient care, enhancing data quality, and addressing health system failures – the third constitutes the inevitable backdrop to transnational medical research under current global economic-political conditions: one of inequality and injustice. Although this level of challenge is beyond simple solutions, an awareness of it – and understanding of its contradictions – is crucial to provide orientation, direction, and thrust to ethical action.

FACILITATOR'S PREPARATION TEMPLATE:

1. Choose a training case study (TCS) suited to your context.
2. What is the key take-home message or learning aim I want to convey to my training participants?
3. What are my secondary learning objectives? Do these include any potential action points?
4. What is the desired outcome of this training exercise, what do I want to achieve?
5. Are there any risks that might jeopardize our discussions? What can I do to avoid potential bottlenecks, or red herrings? Are there possible dead ends in the discussion?
6. What format will the training exercise take?

Key message/Learning objectives:

____

____

____

____

Potential action points:

____

____

____

____

Steps I need to take to achieve the learning outcome and potential action points:

____

____

____

____

FIRST EXPERIENCES OF PILOTING THIS TOOL IN AFRICA AND EUROPE

When we piloted selected case studies and related stories from this workbook with audiences in a number of collaborative African research sites, they were met with astonishing resonance, triggering animated discussions and conversations, and more than one participant remarked plainly how good it was to talk. Supportive remarks and requests for copies of PowerPoint slides went well beyond reactions to ordinary social science presentations.

During piloting, cases were selected after consultation with local scientists. For example, a case on per diems during conferences was removed from the presentation in a site where such per diem rates were under controversial revision. At another site, however, this case study proved to be very constructive: diverse solutions were discussed and dismissed – should employers simply pay hotel bills and not pay per diems? (Laughter; 'No!'); should the conference next time be held in a cheap rural guesthouse? (Hesitation; some acknowledge enjoying 'posh' hotels, others call for 'African' conferences). Discussing the 'Helping hand' case on researchers working in a public hospital with a gathering of healthcare professionals yielded suggestions for improved communication and organization, provoked the formulation of concrete claims to address lack of specific resources in the hospital, and initiated the first ever discussion between the hospital and the wider community about external research in a site that collaborated for two decades. Discussing the story about a Northern graduate student who took on extra consultancy work, on the other hand, gave some expatriate junior researchers a chance to acknowledge and reflect on their co-operation with senior African colleagues, and question their assumptions and role.

While the case studies helped to articulate experiences and release tensions in African research sites, when we piloted them among students and academics in Northern research institutions, they also provided concrete information about how ethical issues play out in real-life situations. This helped those present to understand the challenges arising when 'ethics hit the ground', and served as a source of knowledge about real-life dimensions of global health research, which many of the participants had not yet had a chance to engage with, and which senior academics did not encounter during their short visits to the field. As such, the cases also served as 'ethnographic' data of sorts.

The discussions triggered by the cases did not solve problems, but made it possible to talk about 'awkwardness' in a safe space, giving room to consider potential solutions. Speaking out about inequality can be embarrassing or confrontational, depending on one's position and interlocutors, but it helps those working together across inequality to avoid a sense of merely 'performing' equality, and can build trust, shared visions of collaboration, and joint scientific aims. The greatest danger we identified during the piloting, however, was not confrontation; tensions are not generated by discussion, but ultimately released. Instead, what has to be avoided is participants going away with a sense of futility. At least some elements of steps forward should be identified for further consideration, even if radical and definite solutions do not gain consensus or might seem unrealistic. It is thus important that facilitators consider some possible practical steps in their preparation.

RESOURCES

ETHICS GUIDES AND TOOLKITS

Beskow, L.M. and McCall, J. (Eds). *Informed Consent. Rethinking clinical trials: a living textbook of pragmatic clinical trials.* NIH Health Care Systems Research Collaboratory. Available at: http://sites.duke.edu/rethinkingclinicaltrials/informed-consent-in-pragmatic-clinical-trials (accessed 25 October 2015).

Council for International Organizations of Medical Sciences (2002) CIOMS Guidelines. Available at: http://www.cioms.ch/publications/guidelines/guidelines_nov_2002_blurb.htm (accessed 25 October 2015).

Danis, M. et al (2012) *Research Ethics Consultation: A Casebook,* Oxford University Press USA, New York, New York.

World Health Organization (2009) *Casebook on Ethical Issues in International Health Research.* Available at: http://www.who.int/rpc/publications/ethics_casebook/en/ (accessed 25 October 2015).

World Health Organization (2009) *Research ethics committees: basic concepts for capacity-building.* Available at: http://www.who.int/ethics/Ethics_basic_concepts_ENG.pdf (accessed 25 October 2015).

What journalists want from scientists and why: http://www.scidev.net/global/communication/practical-guide/what-journalists-want-from-scientists-and-why.html (accessed 25 October 2015).

Explaining controversial issues to the media and the public: http://www.scidev.net/global/communication/practical-guide/explaining-controversial-issues-to-the-media-and-t.html (accessed 25 October 2015).

How do I become media savvy? http://www.scidev.net/global/communication/practical-guide/how-do-i-become-media-savvy-.html?from=related%20articles (accessed 25 October 2015).

WEBSITES

The Global Health Network: a massive range of resources to support researchers including a dedicated Global Health Bioethics community site with articles, discussions and e-learning tools. Available at: https://tghn.org/ (accessed 25 October 2015).

Free online training on the protection of human research participants from the National Institute of Health (USA): available at: https://phrp.nihtraining.com/users/login.php (accessed 25 October 2015).

Ongoing consultations in the area of data sharing: Bioethics, Research Ethics & Review. The ethics of data sharing. Available at: https://globalhealthreviewers.tghn.org/community/blogs/post/988/2013/11/the-ethics-of-data-sharing/ (accessed 25 October 2015).

Online tutorial on informed consent: available at: http://www.research.umn.edu/consent/ (accessed 25 October 2015).

JOURNALS

Developing World Bioethics http://eu.wiley.com/WileyCDA/WileyTitle/productCd-DEWB.html (accessed 25 October 2015)

Social Science and Medicine http://www.journals.elsevier.com/social-science-and-medicine/(accessed 25 October 2015)

Bioethics http://onlinelibrary.wiley.com/journal/10.1111/%28ISSN%291467-8519 (accessed 25 October 2015

PART TWO: ACADEMIC BACKGROUND

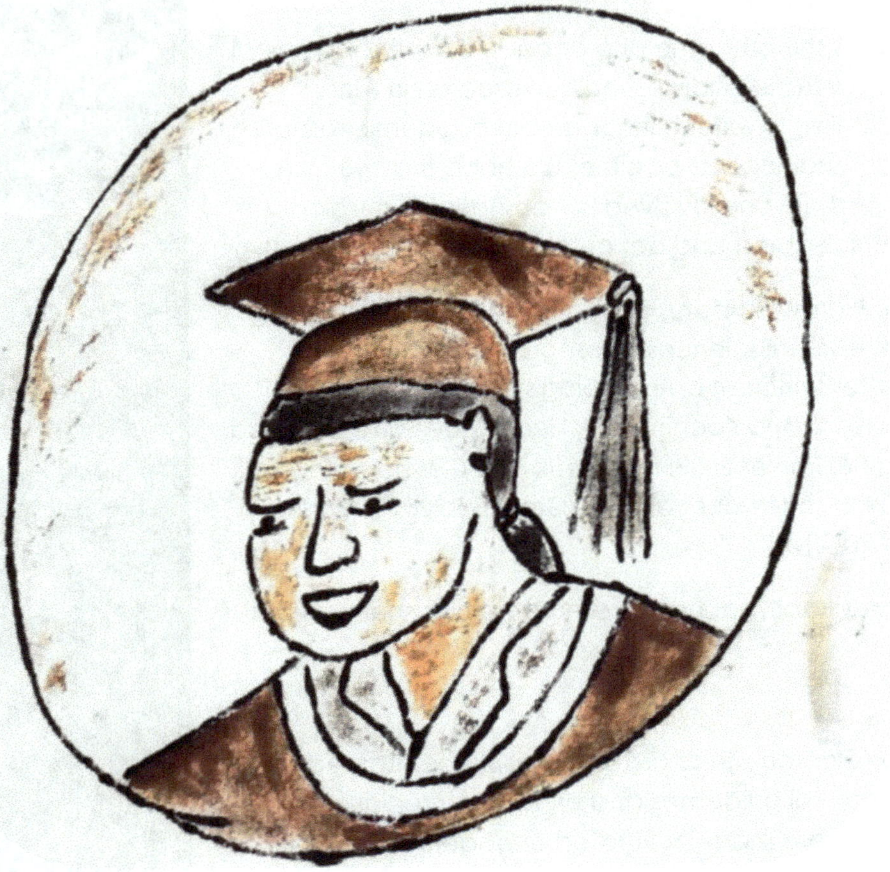

AND NOW FOR THE ANTHROPOLOGY BIT

ACADEMIC BACKGROUND:

ETHICAL DELIBERATION, ENGAGED CONSCIENCE, AND CONSCIOUS CHOICE

This workbook is the outcome of a decade of anthropological studies into how transnational medical research in Africa is carried out. It aims to extend insights from academic research to as wide an audience as possible. We hope that we can thereby support anyone involved in transnational medical research to think about and act on ethical challenges.

Our workbook draws impetus from a growing interest among the qualitative social sciences in research ethics, and increasing attention from anthropologists in particular (for example Marshall and Koenig 2000; Hedgecoe 2004; Fairhead et al 2005, 2006; Parker 2007; Molyneux and Geissler 2008; Simpson 2009; Bandewar et al 2010; Graboyes 2010; Geissler 2011; Whyte 2014).

Anthropological approaches to research ethics share several key ideas:

Ethics happen in practice

While research ethics are (and should be) framed by international guidelines and principles, crucial ethical decisions are made in situated engagements and face-to-face encounters, giving rise to what can be called a 'relational ethics'. These relational ethics cannot replace, but complement and interact with, formal regulatory guidelines and rules.

(See, for example, Kleinman 1999; Molyneux et al 2005; Geissler et al 2008; Gikonyo et al 2008)

KEY LESSONS

Ethics happen in practice.

Ethical situations involve a diversity of actors and arenas.

Research ethics cannot be separated from the economic context of global health research.

There are blind spots and public secrets in research.

Ethical situations involve a diversity of actors and arenas

While research ethics must be guaranteed by public scientific institutions, and hold investigators accountable, many important ethical decisions are taken by technicians and fieldworkers. These 'interface' actors are often considered unproblematic quasi-technical staff; they do not feature prominently in academic publications, nor in research ethics debates. We believe this is a major oversight.

(See, for example, Fairhead et al 2005; Kelly 2011; Benatar and Brock 2011; Molyneux et al 2013; Kamuya 2013; Molyneux, Kamuya et al 2013)

Research ethics cannot be separated from the economic context of global research

Under conditions of widespread deprivation and increasing economic inequality, ethics, economics and politics cannot be separated. Material realities dictate ethical possibilities, and ethics are political. Ethical challenges in transnational research arise not only in relation to vulnerable participants, but also from collaborative and institutional engagements.

(See, for example, Rajan 2005; Petryna 2009; Seth 2009; Rottenburg 2009)

There are blind spots and 'public secrets' in transnational medical research

Due to institutional structures and procedures, everyday ethical challenges experienced by individual actors often receive no attention in research planning and implementation, nor in reporting and publication.

(See, for example, Farmer and Gastineau Campos 2004; Wendland 2010Geissler 2013)

Ethics and structural violence

The authors of this book relate to ongoing discussions among professional bioethicists, especially the concept of 'structural violence'[1] – the idea that the unequal distribution of people's chances to survive, attain or maintain health, develop desirable life courses, or pursue better futures constitutes an underlying injustice (Pogge 2002; Lavery et al 2007; Panitch 2013). In our view, practitioners who daily confront the suffering caused by such inequality have an obligation to try to make a difference, not necessarily to solve entrenched problems but to aim for some sort of improvement (Pogge 2002). In transnational medical research,

[1] This term, borrowed from political science, refers to social structures or institutions which prevent people from meeting their basic needs, and thus harm them without necessarily deploying outright force (see Farmer 2004; Farmer et al. 2006).

which operates across major differences in health, wealth and opportunity, both these injustices and the resulting responsibilities can be particularly painful to deal with.

A systemic perspective

Our position resonates with what ethicists have referred to as 'systemic' perspective: one which situates medical concerns within wider questions of justice, rather than relying on individual doctor-patient relationships to seek improvements. This means viewing the entire field of inequality surrounding transnational research as a *'skandalon'* – not a 'scandal' which calls for clamour and exposition (although there is a place for that, too), but, in the literal sense of the ancient Greek word, a 'stumbling stone' which helps us to stop, seek orientation, and redirect our efforts. This implies an ethics of opening, rather than of regulatory closure. Contrary to ethical arguments which seek to delimit ethical responsibility as a simple matter of scientific 'good practice' – what some critics refer to as a 'minimalist' position (London 2006) – we believe that global inequalities should, indeed, worry transnational medical researchers persistently (Emanuel et al 2005). The first step in any attempt to address system-level inequalities must be to engage one's 'conscience', taking note of larger and smaller stumbling-blocks and the personal challenge which these pose to each of us.

Ethical deliberation

At the same time, research ethics is, for us, less about 'doing the right thing' than about coming to grips with what is wrong. To do this, individuals and groups must develop an ability to express and confront overarching conditions and contradictions, to negotiate agreements about direction and purpose, to seek allies and identify obstacles, and to be open to disagreement and failure. Such debate, which has no easy solutions but encompasses multiple perspectives, has been called 'deliberation'. We follow the argument made by, among others, Gracia (2003), that moral decisions must take into account not only principles and ideas, but also emotions, values and beliefs.

Deliberation is the process in which everyone concerned by the decision is considered a valid moral agent, obliged to give reasons for their own points of view, and to listen to the reasons of others. The goal of this process is not the reaching of a consensus but the enrichment of one's own point of view with that of the others, increasing in this way the maturity of one's own decision, in order to make it wiser or prudent. The people involved in deliberating the case may have different opinions as to how the issues should be resolved, but debating the issues will help change their perceptions of the problem. This is the benefit of the deliberation process.

The case stories in this book invite such deliberation, by prompting positioned and engaged conversation about ethical challenges in context. This, we believe, will enhance our awareness of how global inequalities translate into the minutiae of transnational medical research.

Conscious choices and possibilities

We also hope it will also create awareness of the possibilities which concrete situations and resources provide. Negotiating these possibilities is a matter of making conscious choices, which take into account the inevitable overlapping ethical demands, the limits of catch-all guidelines, any particular resource constraints, and the persistence of wider areas of doubt. This, hopefully, will help practitioners attain the best possible outcome in a given situation.

Seeking the 'best possible' outcome does not, however, mean abandoning ambition. For example, the most radical demands put forth in the late 1990s discussion about standards of HIV care in transnational HIV research in Africa have still not been met; yet the articulation of claims, which many denounced as utopian pipe dreams at the time, has very effectively raised ethical standards. This has meant concrete, material improvements in the treatment of people with HIV, as well as a greater sensitivity to medical justice across the North/South divide across the board. The HIV treatment debate demonstrates that demands which critics denounce as 'impossible' may, in fact, reflect only mundane obstacles such as funding limitations, time constraints, or a lack of political will. If, therefore, activists today demand that research organizations help to establish functioning in-country public healthcare systems, we cannot simply dismiss such claims offhand as 'unrealistic' (de Cenival 2008).

While such radical demands (which call, in effect, for public health research to act as a tool in overarching social transformation) must be taken seriously, they are not always directly useful on the ground. The focus of this book is not to make any such case. Rather, we seek to empower specific agents to create small-scale improvements, making the most of contextual opportunities and alliances. At the same time, if working with this book prompts the collective insight that we can do more – indeed, that we persistently *must* do more, rather than sit comfortably with minimal ethical arrangements – new directions might take hold in research culture. This may, eventually, lead to a wider engagement of medical research with the political context of systemic problems. This, we believe, is a goal worth striving for.

THE CONTEXT OF GLOBAL HEALTH INEQUALITY

Due to the particular experience of the authors of this book, our starting-point is medical research conducted by African, European and North American institutions in Africa, but we hope that the book will be useful in relation to research in other economically deprived societies (Rajan 2005; Petryna 2009; Abadie, 2010; Meyers and Hunt 2014). The main challenges to health and wellbeing is global political, economic, and epidemiological inequality, as well as unequal possibilities. While these issues recur in many contexts, the African continent offers some particularly stark patterns of difference (e.g. Prince and Marsland 2013; Geissler 2013, 2014b).

Adverse medical, economic and political conditions in Africa are historically produced, and shaped by the legacy of colonialism. This is evident in the many echoes of 'imperial science' (e.g. Clarke 2007; Giles-Vernick and Webb 2013; Manton 2013) which persist in today's research. Like the research conducted in Africa by imperial regimes, transnational research today operates across huge differentials in power, resources, and knowledge, and involves global circulations and transfers of personnel and expertise, apparatus and techniques, and data. Expressions such as 'overseas research', or 'going out' or 'going down' to African sites (even when these units are located in major capital cities), continue to express hierarchical centre-periphery geographies, implying secluded islands of civilization in the wilderness.

Using such language sends a clear message to African scientific colleagues about their subservient relationship to Northern institutions, despite any claims in other contexts to 'equal collaboration', and it suggests that conceptual maps of power have altered little in the transition from colonialism to post-colonialism. It is all too easy for apparently extinct ethical positions to creep in alongside such world-views.

The persistence of these terms also highlights that ill health and poverty are not simply technical problems, but are grounded in historically shaped inequality – the deprivation of large groups of people, in relation to others, through ongoing global processes. While the actual geography of deprivation has changed somewhat, so that inequality appears increasingly between a global middle class and the vast majority, rather than between countries, the basic problem remains. Relative ill health is not a remediable accident, but a direct outcome of the relationships between more and less affluent people.

With this in view, this workbook aims to support 'public' transnational health research – scientific work which is predominantly funded by public institutions, is conducted by publicly employed scientists, shares its results in the public domain, and aims at public health improvements. It is important to differentiate such public research from rapidly growing for-profit medical research, such as that conducted by pharmaceutical and genomics institutions, often through transnational 'contract research organizations' (Petryna 2007; Foster and Malik 2012). In many cases, such research views global inequality as a condition for profit maximization rather than social good. Public medical research, by contrast, is at least partly directed towards social justice, with its actors motivated by the struggle against the effects of inequality on health and wellbeing.

Public medical research is, like science and academia more generally, under threat from particular economic and political interests. For example, pharmaceutical companies influence research agendas in order to open up markets for new vaccines, to gain knowledge for drugs directed at Northern customers, or to gain public trust and tax relief. And research funded by Northern governments into the 'tropical' diseases of the poor also usefully protects the military in overseas operations. Northern 'security' agendas, for example those related to emergent viral diseases, can overwrite an older public health impetus grounded in international solidarity and basic needs.

At the same time, consortia and public-private partnerships such as the HIV Prevention Trials Network (HPTN) or the GAVI alliance, which emphasize technical fixes like vaccines and drugs, make use of private funding and expertise. On the one hand this can enhance the speed and scope of public health interventions, but on the other it can jeopardize scientific independence and introduce industry influences into the public domain (Jain 2013). In the face of these threats to public medical research, it is of particular importance to retain the analytic distinction between public and private science.

Transnational medical research has been expanding over the past few decades (Petryna 2009). Global institutions and consortia are conducting growing numbers of trials, connecting more and more researchers through collaborations across geographic, cultural, and economic divides. Such work is often conducted under the remit of fairly durable institutional agreements, and in sites which attract substantial investment in infrastructure and human resources (Gerrets 2014; Okwaro and Geissler 2015). Many of these powerful and well-endowed collaborations have achieved a quasi-permanent existence through consecutive funding, with a lasting physical presence. Personnel, too, often look to running employment, even if on renewable annual contracts.

These highly productive research sites harbour particular challenges, because they juxtapose the radically different medical and scientific possibilities of local and international actors, and bring into confrontation diverse personal motivations and lifestyles. But because of the quality of scientific work they permit, and because of their size and long-term prospects, they also offer opportunities to lay the foundations for more sustainable national and regional scientific institutions, and continuous public health improvements. Successful collaborations create a wide range of relations which evolve over time, allowing not only for scientific discovery and progress, but also for the growth and development of personal relationships. In turn, hopefully, this can produce even better science. It is especially this process of long-term scientific engagement across difference to which our workbook hopes to make a modest contribution.

INEQUALITY AND DISCOMFORT

Inequality shapes the field of transnational medical research in at least three key ways:

Firstly, unequal economic conditions result in exposure to pathogens and cause malnutrition; the resulting infectious diseases remain the focus of transnational medical research. The entire field depends upon the fight against such 'diseases of poverty' for its legitimizing discourse.

Secondly, underfunded and weak post-colonial healthcare infrastructures, and a concomitant lack of drugs, diagnostics, qualified staff, and technology, are a crucial factor in most transnational projects. They drive researchers to come up with new interventions, but they also limit research in that they require tools which can operate alongside malfunctioning healthcare systems (Redfield 2008; Lancet 2009; Biehl and Petryna 2013; Geissler 2014b). Weak public health systems also have an impact on informed consent in recruitment, and on data validity; and they shape the experience and motivations of health practitioners and scientists working in research (Crane 2010).

Thirdly, inequality in transnational medical research pertains to scientific knowledge itself, and the conditions of its production. Neglected for decades by national governments and overseas agencies, universities and scientific institutions in many Southern countries have fallen far behind Northern institutions in terms of scientific expertise, output, and recognition. Their ability to produce innovative and generalizable scientific knowledge has been severely limited.

These domains of gross inequality, pertaining to health and wellbeing and to education and knowledge, remain a persistent provocation to public health science. Even advocates of free-market policies usually find it difficult to contest the fundamental human right to health and to knowledge. Since the ethics of transnational medical research is centred around inequality, it is hard to differentiate it from the *politics* of medical research: the legitimate interests, contests and struggles which occur within and around medical research settings – between researchers and research participants, funders and scientists, or institutions and researchers of different origins. This is why we chose to include the notion of 'political' deliberation into the remit of this book, to retain a prominent place for reflections on power, structural violence and contested interests. It is one of the premises of our work that ethical reflection which aims to steer free of political-economic questions, externalizing these as being 'beyond research', ultimately leaves unaddressed the most central choices which have to be taken in the pursuit of medical science and public health progress (see Kleinman 1999; Farmer and Gastineau Campos 2004; Geissler 2013).

The ethics of transnational medical research, then, can only ever aim to 'do the right thing' within a wrong global and local order; and under such conditions, in fact, it is impossible to identify beyond doubt and for once and for all, what is 'right'. As illustrated by the conundra presented in this book, this makes for an essentially 'uncomfortable' position (Lavery et al 2010, 2013), which rarely allows for stable settlements, fixed rules, or even obvious good practice. Such discomfort should lead neither to nihilism, nor to over-ambitious demands which can have a paralysing or divisive effect if lacking a basis in current political realities. A sense of discomfort, instead, could provoke ongoing critical reflection, helping practitioners to figure out the best options in a particular situation and to create incremental improvements – while remaining aware of the fragility of such attempts. This workbook, therefore, does not aim to prevent its readers from feeling uncomfortable.

EMERGENT DEBATES

The less-than-straightforward nature of the ethical challenges, the lack of clear and lasting solutions, and the indeterminate mode of progress driven by the type of critical engagement we are advocating, is evident in the history of transnational medical research ethics over the past two decades.

The 'standards of care' controversy

To many, this history starts with the late 1990s 'standards of care' controversy around HIV research in Africa (Angell 1997, 2000; Lurie and Wolf 1997; Wendland 2008). At the core of this acrimonious debate was outrage about the fact that African research participants in trials of a cheap and simple (though presumably less efficacious) drug regime to prevent HIV transmission from mother to child, received a placebo as comparison rather than the standard North American treatment, which relied on expensive drugs and health facilities, and was at the time unavailable in Africa. When these concerns were first raised around 1997, some of our colleagues involved in these attempts to develop effective, low-cost interventions against the spread of HIV in Africa were aggrieved. What did the critics hope to achieve? How could time-limited individual projects be asked to fill gaps in the public health system? What funder would be willing to pay additional costs of US-standard treatment and monitoring? How could one develop 'adapted' healthcare interventions, feasible under prevalent conditions in Africa, if ethicists insisted in applying global standards of care (Bhutta et al 2004)?

Both sides in this debate grew heated. Some did not shy away from evocative comparisons with the US experiments at Tuskegee, or even Nazi experimentation. Others, in turn, accused the critics of killing HIV positive Africans by preventing the timely development of appropriate and realistic treatment and prevention. The controversy was fueled by the combatants' personal stakes in HIV research, while Northern HIV activism framed HIV as a rights issue rather than a public health emergency (see Fisher et al, 2009). Some measures were taken which now seem mistaken, including the closure of important trials.

In one sense the debate fell far too short: 15 years later, no consensus has been reached about how to bridge the standards of care in the Northern medical institutions, in which trials are often designed, and the Southern healthcare systems in which they are conducted (Feierman 2011). Yet while this affair did not bring about the dramatic change which radical critics had hoped for, it did engender momentous shifts. For one, the confrontations raised awareness about the deficiency of regulations at the time, leading to innovations such as the concept of 'good clinical practice' and the establishment of ethical review boards.

The regulatory turn

The introduction of improved regulation was an important step in the development of transnational medical research ethics. Yet some critics have pointed out that these changes have had their own negative consequences (see e.g. Farmer and Gastineau Campos 2004). Taking into perspective the issues of wider injustice described above, regulation can appear to proclaim overly simply solutions, ignoring local entanglements. The regulatory emphasis on informed consent can seem to focus too much on research participants' autonomy, instead of on mutual obligations between researchers and participants. In emphasizing participants' individual, discrete choices, without exploring the wider context, some accuse the consent process of intentionally obscuring the wider conditions which create ill health.

Ethical rulebooks can also foster a culture of superficial compliance, behind which nihilism can persist (Lachenal 2015). As illustrated in some of the case studies in this workbook, 'ethics' in this particular sense can silence debate, rather than foster it: if 'consent' is taken to be a participant's signature, obtained as quickly as possible, then consensual engagement fades from view. If guidelines forbid material remuneration, then payments to research participants may be knowingly mislabelled as 'transport reimbursement' (Geissler 2011b). If an ethics review board chairman uses the ironic question 'So you want to change the African health system?' to silence board members' questions about post-trial care, then the whole process risks becoming a rubberstamping procedure.

And yet, some hard and fast rules are needed. The 'ethical minimalism' of relying solely on regulation constitutes a universal ethical baseline which can hold to account more 'relational practices' based on individual conscience. Under conditions of marked inequality, without regulation personal relations can easily be manipulated to serve specific interests. Even if these support a scientific goal, this would compromise informed consent and data validity. Moreover, in the absence of definite rules, ad-hoc decisions can more easily be taken by senior Principal Investigators and grant holders than by local frontline staff, which is both inequitable and reduces efficiency. Regulation has a role in granting agency and a certain form of transparency to all involved. Its overall value must depend, of course, on how it is implemented.

Overall, the overseas bioethics discussion has opened a new space for deliberation, ranging all the way from issues of individual patient care to structural questions of institutional inequality. On the one hand, regulatory minimalists seek to prevent abuse through general and enforceable rules, while on the other, activists articulate ambitious demands, seeking to make public health research a tool in overarching social transformation. This debate has continued to develop precisely because simple and lasting solutions are not easily found. It has led to more nuanced reflections on what constitutes a legitimate ethical concern: for example, the initial outrage about HIV treatment has led on to questions over participants' rights to sustained antiretroviral treatment after projects end. Increasing numbers of trials now provide this, as well as healthcare beyond the immediate focus of their research. Even where provision is more basic, the debates have provided a vocabulary of claims for trial participants and their advocates. The reliance of HIV prevention trials on continued exposure, too – most notably in so-called 'high-risk' groups – has come under scrutiny. Here, the intimate relation between medical research and the social context on which it is predicated is particularly evident.

A changing ethical landscape in medical research

Increased ethical sensitivity in transnational medical research has widened beyond HIV. For example, the Neglected Disease Initiative promotes research into treatments for diseases of the poor which do not promise profits for the pharmaceutical industry (Allen and Parker 2012). Bioethics debates have also emerged around the ownership of value generated from biological specimens, for example in genomics research, the storage of specimens, and the distribution of benefits (Chokshi et al 2006). Discussion around bioethics in research has led to renewed emphasis on capacity building, and obliged Northern initiatives to invest further in involving African people in research, sometimes as a funding requirement (Chu et al 2014).[2] While all these provisions can be circumvented or used as 'fig leaves', they nonetheless point in the right direction.

Gradually, and with inevitable setbacks, wrong turns and conflicts, bioethics discussions have changed the landscape of medical research. In 1994 Geissler could, as a PhD student, collect blood from schoolchildren without individual or parental consent, legitimized purely by the national government's Ministries of Health and Education. Six years later, a major research project in the same area was closed prematurely after the United States-based evaluators found that no individual written consent had been obtained. Again, many of these moves risk becoming atrophied and turned into meaningless rituals; they can be kept vital only through continuous debate. We believe that these deliberations will, little by little, change the daily practices of transnational medical research for the better.

---

[2] At the end of colonialism such efforts were labelled 'Africanization'. The persistence of the term in discussions of research provides yet another point of continuity between the past, present, and suggested future of medical research in Africa.

WE NEED TO TALK MORE; WE NEED TO DO MORE

This workbook was initially titled *'We need to talk more'* – a phrase that came up during a public discussion with staff at a large health research station in Africa about the challenges of everyday scientific fieldwork. The speaker meant that staff would benefit from talking more about issues that seemingly were either too obvious, too personal or contentious, or too irresolvable, to be spoken about in professional conversations across divides in disciplinary training, hierarchical position, and origin. Talking remains, however, just the first step: when we more recently presented a draft of this workbook in an African research laboratory, somebody suggested that we change the title to *'We need to do more'*.

We hope this workbook might be a small catalyst for translating talk into action. Discussing the tensions which arise from the endeavours of public health actors to 'do the right thing', and to combat some of the effects of entrenched global injustice, will not make the latter go away. But it might help to sharpen the tools here and there, allowing us to identify what we need to do in order to make improvements in our individual settings. Inspired by all those engaged in transnational medical research who believe that their efforts will eventually lead to better global health, the social scientists behind this book hope to empower practitioners to develop their own, relationally engaged approaches to ethical practice, which may one day, in turn, contribute to increased social justice.

REFERENCES

Aellah, G. and Geissler, P.W (2016) Seeking exposure: conversions of scientific knowledge in an African City: *Journal of Modern African Studies*, 54(3) pp 389-417

Abadie, R. (2010) *The Professional Guinea Pig: Big Pharma and the Risky World of Human Subjects.* Duke University Press, Durham, North Carolina.

Allen, T. and Parker, M. (2012) Will increased funding for neglected tropical diseases really make poverty history? *The Lancet* 379(9821), 1097–1098.

Angell, M. (1997) The ethics of clinical research in the Third World. *New England Journal of Medicine* 337, 853–856.

Angell, M. (2000) Investigators' responsibilities for human subjects in developing countries. *New England Journal of Medicine* 342, 967–969.

Angweniyi, V. et al. (2014) Complex realities: community engagement for a paediatric randomized controlled malaria vaccine trial in Kilifi, Kenya. Trials 15, 65. DOI: 10.1186/1745-6215-15-65.

April, M. (2010) Rethinking HIV exceptionalism: the ethics of opt-out HIV testing in sub-Saharan Africa. *Bulletin of the World Health Organization* 88, 703–708. DOI: 10.2471/BLT.09.073049 Available at: http://www.who.int/bulletin/volumes/88/9/09-073049/en/ (accessed 25 October 2015).

Bandewar, S., Kimani, J. et al. (2010) The origins of a research community in the Majengo observational cohort study, Nairobi, Kenya. *BMC Public Health* 10(1), 1–10.

Bell, K. and Elliott, D. (2014) Censorship in the name of ethics: critical public health research in the age of human subjects regulation. *Critical Public Health* 24(4): 385 - 391.

Benatar, S.R. and Singer, P.A. (2010) Responsibilities in international research: a new look revisited. *Journal of Medical Ethics* 36(4), 194–197.

Benatar, S.R. and Brock, G. (eds) (2011) *Global Health and Global Health Ethics.* Cambridge University Press, Cambridge, UK.

Beskow, L.M. and McCall, J. (Eds). *Informed Consent. Rethinking clinical trials: a living textbook of pragmatic clinical trials.* NIH Health Care Systems Research Collaboratory. Available at:

http://sites.duke.edu/rethinkingclinicaltrials/informed-consent-in-pragmatic-clinical-trials (accessed 25 October 2015).

Bhutta, Z. (2004) Standards of care in research. *British Medical Journal* 329(7475), 1114–1115.

Biehl, J. and Petryna, A. (2013) *When People Come First: Critical Studies in Global Health*. Princeton University Press, Princeton, New Jersey.

Brown, H. (2015) Global health partnerships, governance, and sovereign responsibility in western Kenya. *American Ethnologist* 42, 340–355. doi:10.1111/amet.12134

Carrel, M. and Rennie, S. (2008) Demographic and health surveillance: longitudinal ethical considerations. *Bulletin of the World Health Organization* 86(8), 612–616.

Caulfield, T. (2005) Legal and ethical issues associated with patient recruitment in clinical trials: the case of competitive enrolment. *Health Law Review* 13(2–3), 58–61.

de Cenival, M. (2008) L'éthique de la recherche ou la liberté d'en sortir. *Bulletin of the Exotic Pathology Society* 101(2), 98–101.

Chantler, T., Otewa, F. et al. (2013) Ethical challenges that arise at the community interface of health research: village reporters' experiences in Western Kenya. *Developing World Bioethics* 13(1), 30–37.

Chokshi, D.A., Parker, M., and Kwiatkowski, D.P. (2006) Data sharing and intellectual property in a genomic epidemiology network: policies for large-scale research collaboration. *Bulletin of the World Health Organization* 84(5), 382–387.

Chu, K.M., Jayaraman, S., Kyamanywa, P., and Ntakiyiruta, G. (2014) Building research capacity in Africa: equity and global health collaborations. *PloS Med* 11(3), e1001612. DOI: 10.1371/journal.pmed.1001612

Clarke, S. (2007) A technocratic imperial state? The colonial office and scientific research, 1940–1960. *Twentieth Century British History* 18(4), 453–480.

Conteh, L. and Kingori, P. (2010) Per diems in Africa: a counter-argument. *Tropical Medicine & International Health* 15(12), 1553–1555.

Cooper, M. (2013) Double exposure – sex workers, biomedical prevention trials, and the dual logic of global public health. *Scholar and Feminist Online* 11(3), 1–11.

Corneli, A.L. et al. (2012) Improving participant understanding of informed consent in an HIV-prevention clinical trial: a comparison of methods. *Aids and Behaviour* 16(2), 412–421.

REFERENCES

Council for International Organizations of Medical Sciences (2002) CIOMS Guidelines. Available at: http://www.cioms.ch/publications/guidelines/guidelines_nov_2002_blurb.htm (accessed 25 October 2015).

Crane, J.T. (2010) Unequal 'partners': AIDS, academia and the rise of global health. *Behemoth* 3, 78–97. DOI: http://dx.doi.org/10.1524/behe.2010.0021

Crane, J.T. (2011) Scrambling for Africa? Universities and global health. *The Lancet* 377(9775), 1388–1390.

Crane, J.T. (2013) *Scrambling for Africa: AIDS, expertise, and the rise of American global health science*. Cornell University Press, Ithaca, New York.

Diallo, D.A., Doumbo, O.K., Plowe, C.V., Wellems, T.E., Emanuel, E.J., and Hurst, S.A. (2005) Community permission for medical research in developing countries. *Clinical Infectious Diseases* 41, 255–259.

Emanuel, E.J., Wendler, D., Killen, J., and Grady, C. (2004) What makes clinical research in developing countries ethical? The benchmarks of ethical research. *Journal of Infectious Disease* 189, 930–937.

Emanuel, E. J., Currie, X.E. et al. (2005) Undue inducement in clinical research in developing countries: is it a worry? *The Lancet* 366(9482), 336–340.

Fairhead, J., Leach, M. et al. (2005). Public engagement with science? Local understandings of a vaccine trial in The Gambia. *Journal of Biosocial Science*, 38(1): 103-116.

Fairhead, J., Leach, M., and Small, M. (2006) Where techno-science meets poverty: medical research and the economy of blood in The Gambia, West Africa. *Social Science and Medicine* 63(4), 1109–1120.

Farmer, P. (2004) An anthropology of structural violence. *Current Anthropology* 45(3), 305–325.

Farmer, P. and Gastineau Campos, N. (2004) New malaise: bioethics and human rights in the global era. *Journal of Law, Medicine & Ethics* 32, 243–251.

Farmer, P.E., Nizeye, B., Stulac, S., and Keshavjee, S. (2006) Structural violence and clinical medicine. *PLoS Medicine* 3(10), e449. http://doi.org/10.1371/journal.pmed.0030449

Feierman, S. (2011) When physicians meet: local medical knowledge and global public goods. In: Geissler, P. and Molyneux, C. (eds.) *Evidence, Ethos and Ethnography: The Anthropology and History of Medical Research in Africa*. Berghahn, Oxford, UK, pp. 171–196.

Feldman-Savelsberg, P., Ndonko, F.T., and Schmidt-Ehry, B. (2000) Sterilizing vaccines or the politics of the womb: retrospective study of a rumor in Cameroon. *Medical Anthropology Quarterly* 14, 159–179.

Fisher, W., Kohut, T., Fischer, J. (2009) AIDS exceptionalism: on the social psychology of HIV prevention research. *Social Issues Policy Review* 3(1), 45–77.

Foster, C. and Malik, A.Y. (2012) The elephant in the (board) room: the role of contract research organizations in international clinical research. *The American Journal of Bioethics* 12(11), 49–50.

Geissler, P.W. (2005) 'Kachinja are coming!': encounters around medical research work in a Kenyan village. *Africa: Journal of the International African Institute* 75, 173–202.

Geissler, P.W. (2011). Studying trial communities: anthropological and historical inquiries into ethos, politics and economy of medical research in Africa. In: Geissler, P. and Molyneux, C. (eds.) *Evidence, Ethos and Ethnography: The Anthropology and History of Medical Research in Africa*. Berghahn, Oxford, UK, pp. 1–28.

Geissler, P.W. (2011) 'Transport to where?': reflections on the problem of value and time *à propos* an awkward practice in medical research. *Journal of Cultural Economy* 4(1) 45 -64.

Geissler, P.W. (2013) Public secrets in public health: knowing not to know while making scientific knowledge. *American Ethnologist* 40(1), 13–34.

Geissler, P.W. (2013). The archipelago of public health. Comments on the landscape of medical research in twenty-first century Africa. In: Prince, R. and Marsland, R. *Making and Unmaking Public Health in Africa. Ethnographic and Historical Perspectives.* Athens, Ohio University Press: 231-256.

Geissler, P.W. (2013) Stuck in ruins, or up and coming? The shifting geography of urban public health research in Kisumu, Kenya. *Africa: Journal of the International African Institute* 83, 539–560.

Geissler, P.W. (ed) (2014) *Para-states and Medical Science: Making Global Health in Africa.* Duke University Press, Durham, North Carolina.

Geissler, P.W. (2014) Introduction. In: Geissler, W. (ed.) *Para-states and Medical Science: Making Global Health in Africa.* Duke University Press, Durham, North Carolina,1-54.

Geissler, P.W. (2014). What future remains? Remembering an African place of science. In: Geissler, P.W. (ed.) *Para-states and Medical Science: Making Global Health in Africa.* Duke University Press, Durham, North Carolina 142-178.

Geissler, P.W. and Molyneux, C. (eds.) (2011) *Evidence, Ethos and Ethnography: The Anthropology and History of Medical Research in Africa.* Berghahn, Oxford, UK.

Geissler, P.W. and Pool, R. (2006) Editorial: Popular concerns about medical research projects in sub-Saharan Africa – a critical voice in debates about medical research ethics. *Tropical Medicine & International Health* 11(7), 975–982.

Geissler, P.W., Kelly, A., Imoukhuede B., and Pool, R. (2008) 'He is now like a brother, I can even give him some blood' – relational ethics and material exchanges in a malaria vaccine 'trial community' in The Gambia. *Social Science and Medicine* 67(5), 696–707.

Gerrets, R. (2014) International health and the proliferation of 'partnerships': (un)intended boost for state institutions in Tanzania. In: Geissler, W. (ed.) *Para-states and Medical Science: Making Global Health in Africa.* Duke University Press, Durham, North Carolina, pp. 196–206.

Gikonyo, C., Bejon, P. et al. (2008) Taking social relationships seriously: lessons learned from the informed consent practices of a vaccine trial on the Kenyan coast. *Social Science & Medicine* 67(5), 708–720.

Giles-Vernick, T. and Webb, J. (eds.) (2013) *Global Health in Africa: Historical Perspectives on Disease Control.* Ohio University Press, Athens, Ohio.

Global Campaign for Microbicides (2004) *Mobilization for Community Involvement in Microbicides Trials: A Report from a Dialogue in Southern Africa.* Washington DC, USA. Accessed 27th June 2016: http://www.global-campaign.org/clientfiles/SA-community-involvement.pdf

Graboyes, M. (2010) Fines, orders, fears... and consent? Medical research in East Africa c.1950s. *Developing World Bioethics* 10(1), 34–41.

Gracia, D. (2003) Ethical case deliberation and decision making. *Medicine, Health Care and Philosophy* 6(3), 227–233.

Grant, R.W. and Sugarman, J. (2004) Ethics in human subjects research: do incentives matter? *Journal of Medicine and Philosophy* 29(6), 717–738.

Hantel, A., Olopade, CO. (2015) Drug and Vaccine Access in the Ebola Epidemic: Advising Caution in Compassionate Use. *Ann Intern Med* 162, 141-142.

Hedgecoe, A. M. (2004). Critical bioethics: Beyond the social science critique of applied ethics. *Bioethics* 18(2) 120–143.

Irikefe, V. et al. (2011) Science in Africa@ the view from the frontline. Published online 29 June 2011, *Nature* 474, 556-559. Doi: 10.1038/474556a.

Jain, A. (2013) HPV vaccination as a national health priority: no easy answers. *BMJ* 347: f5634.

Jentsch, B. and Pilley C. (2003) Research relationships between the South and the North: Cinderella and the ugly sisters? *Social Science and Medicine* 57, 1957–1967.

Kalofonos, I.A. (2010) 'All I eat is ARVs': the paradox of AIDS treatment interventions in Central Mozambique. *Medical Anthropology Quarterly* 24(3), 363–380.

Kamuya, D., Marsh, V., and Molyneux, S. (2011) What we learned about voluntariness and consent: incorporating 'background situations' and understanding into analyses. *The American Journal of Bioethics* 11(8), 31–33. PubMed PMID: 21806436.

Kamuya, D.M., Theobald, S.J. et al. (2013) Evolving friendships and shifting ethical dilemmas: fieldworkers' experiences in a short term community based study in Kenya. *Developing World Bioethics* 13(1), 1–9.

Kelly, A. (2011) Remember Bambali: evidence, ethics and the co-production of truth. In: Geissler, P.W. and Molyneux, C. (eds.) *Evidence, Ethos and Ethnography: The Anthropology and History of Medical Research in Africa*. Berghahn, Oxford, UK, pp. 229–244.

Kelly, A. (2011) Will he be there? Mediating malaria, immobilizing science. *Journal of Cultural Economy* 4(1), 65–79.

Kelly, A.H. and Wenzel Geissler, P. (2011) Introduction: The value of transnational medical research. *Journal of Cultural Economy* 4(1), 3–10.

Kelly, A.H., Pinder, M., Ameh, D., Majambere, S., and Lindsay, S. (2011) 'Like Sugar and Honey': the embedded ethics of a larval control project in The Gambia. *Social Science & Medicine* 70 (12), 1912–1919.

Kingori, P. (2015) When the science fails and the ethics works: 'Fail-safe' ethics in the FEM-PrEP study. *Anthropology and Medicine* Epub 2015 Oct 20, 1-17

Kingori, P. (2015) The 'empty choice': a sociological examination of choosing medical research participation in resource-limited sub-Saharan Africa. *Current Sociology* 63(5), 763–778.

Kingori, P. et al. (2010) 'Rumours' and clinical trials: a retrospective examination of a paediatric malnutrition study in Zambia, southern Africa. *BMC Public Health* 10(1), 556.

Kithinji, C. and Kass, N.E. (2010) Assessing the readability of non-English-language consent forms: the case of Kiswahili for research conducted in Kenya. *IRB: Ethics & Human Research* 32 (4), 10–15.

Kleinman, A. (1999) Moral experience and ethical reflection: can ethnography reconcile them? A quandary for 'the new bioethics'. *Daedalus* (Special Issue: Bioethics and Beyond), 128(4), 69–97.

Lachenal, G. (2015) Lessons in medical nihilism. Virus hunters, neoliberalism and the AIDS crisis in Cameroon. In: Geissler, P.W. (ed.) *Para-states and medical science: making African global science*. Duke University Press, Durham, North Carolina,103–141.

Lachenal, G., Owona Ntsama, J., Ze Bekolo, D., Kombang Ekodogo, T., Manton, J. (2016) Neglected Actors in Neglected Tropical Diseases Research: Historical Perspectives on Health Workers and Contemporary Buruli Ulcer Research in Ayos, Cameroon. *PLoS Neglected Tropical Disease* 10(4): e0004488. doi:10.1371/journal.pntd. 0004488

Lairumbi, G.M. et al. (2008) Promoting the social value of research in Kenya: examining the practical aspects of collaborative partnerships using an ethical frame. *Social Science and Medicine* 67(5), 734–747.

Lairumbi, G.M. et al. (2011) Ethics in practice: the state of the debate on promoting the social value of global health research in resource-poor settings, particularly Africa. *BMC Medical Ethics* 12(22), 1–8.

Lancet. (2009) Editorial: what has the Gates Foundation done for global health? *The Lancet* 373(9675), 1577.

Lang, T. (2011) Advancing global health research through digital technology and sharing data. *Science* 331(6018), 714–717.

Lavery, J. V., Grady, C. et al. (2007) *Ethical Issues in International Biomedical Research*. Oxford University Press, Oxford, UK.

Larson, H., Cooper, L., Eskola, J., Katz, S., Ratzan, S. (2011) Addressing the Vaccine Confidence Gap. *The Lancet* 378:9790, 526–535

Lavery, J., Bandewar, S. et al. (2010) Relief of oppression: an organizing principle for researchers' obligations to participants in observational studies in the developing world. *BMC Public Health* 10(1), 1–7.

Lavery, J. V., Green, S.K. et al. (2013) Addressing ethical, social, and cultural issues in global health research. *PLoS Neglected Tropical Diseases* 7(8): e2227.

Leach, M. and Fairhead, J. (2011) Being 'with Medical Research Council': infant care and the social meanings of cohort membership in Gambia's plural therapeutic landscapes. In: Geissler, W. and Molyneux, C. (eds.) *Evidence, Ethos and Experiment: The Anthropology and History of Medical Research in Africa*. Berghahn Books, Oxford, UK, pp. 77–98.

Lederman, R. (2007) Comparative "Research": A modest proposal concerning the object of ethics regulation. *PoLAR: Political and Legal Anthropology Review* 30(2): 305-327.

London, A. (2006) What is social and global justice to bioethics or bioethics to social and global justice? *Hastings Center Report* 36, no.4.

Lurie, P. and Wolff, S. (1997) Unethical trials of interventions to reduce perinatal transmission of the human immunodeficiency virus in developing countries. *New England Journal of Medicine* 337, 853–856.

Mack, N., Ramirez, C.B., Friedland, B., and Nnko, S. (2013) Lost in translation: assessing effectiveness of focus group questioning techniques to develop improved translation of terminology used in HIV prevention clinical trials. *PLoS One* 8(9): e73799.

Madiega, P.A., Jones, G. et al. (2013). 'She's my sister-In-law, my visitor, my friend' – challenges of staff identity in home follow-up in an HIV trial in Western Kenya. *Developing World Bioethics* 13(1), 21–29.

Manton, J. (2013) Environmental Akalism and the war on filth: the personification of sanitation in urban Nigeria. *Africa: Journal of the International African Institute* 83, 606–622.

Marsh, V., Kamuya, D., Rowa, Y., Gikonyo, C., and Molyneux, S. (2008) Beginning community engagement at a busy biomedical research programme: experiences from the KEMRI CGMRC-Wellcome Trust Research Programme, Kilifi, Kenya. *Social Science and Medicine 67*, 721–733.

Marsh, V., Kamuya, D., Mlamba, A., Williams, S., Molyneux, S. (2010) Experiences with community engagement and informed consent in a genetic cohort study of severe childhood diseases in Kenya. *BMC Medical Ethics*, 11-13

Marshall, P.A. and Koenig, B.A. (2000) Intersections of bioethics and anthropology: locating the 'good' in medical practice. *Anthropologie et sociétés* 24(2), 35–55.

Meslin, E.M. (2008) Achieving global justice in health through global research ethics: supplementing Macklin's 'top-down' approach with one from the 'ground up'. In: Green, R.M., Donovan, A., and Jauss, S.A. (eds.) *Global Bioethics: Issues of Conscience for the Twenty-First Century*. Clarendon Press, Oxford, UK.

Meyers, T. and Hunt, N.R. (2014) The other global south. *The Lancet*: 384(9958):1921-1922.

Mfutso-Bengo J, Ndebele P. et al. (2008) Why do individuals agree to enrol in clinical trials? A qualitative study of health research participation in Blantyre, Malawi. *Malawi Medical Journal* 20: 37-41.

Mills, E. et al. (2005) Media reporting of tenofovir trials in Cambodia and Cameroon. *BMC International Health and Human Rights* 5(1), 6.

Molyneux, C. S., Peshu, N. et al. (2004) Understanding of informed consent in a low-income setting: three case studies from the Kenyan coast. *Social Science & Medicine* 59(12), 2547–2559.

Molyneux, C.S., Peshu, N. et al. (2005) Trust and informed consent: insights from community members on the Kenyan coast. *Social Science and Medicine* 61(7), 1463–73.

Molyneux, C. S., Wassenaar, D.R. et al. (2005b) 'Even if they ask you to stand by a tree all day, you will have to do it (laughter)...!': community voices on the notion and practice of informed consent for biomedical research in developing countries. *Social Science & Medicine* 61(2), 443–454.

Molyneux, S. and Geissler, P.W. (2008) Ethics and the ethnography of medical research in Africa. *Social Science & Medicine* 67(5), 685–695.

Molyneux, S., Mulupi, S., Mbaabu, L. and Marsh, V. (2012) Benefits and payments for research participants : experiences and views from a research centre on the Kenyan coast. *BMC Medical Ethics* Jun 22, 13:13.

Molyneux, S., Kamuya, D. et al. (2013) Field workers at the interface. *Developing World Bioethics* 13(1), ii–iv.

Molyneux, S. et al. (2013). Introduction: Field Workers at the Interface. *Developing World Bioethics* 13(1): ii-iv.

Mondain, N. (2010) Exploring respondents' understanding and perceptions of demographic surveillance systems in Western Africa: methodological and ethical issues. *African Population Studies* 24(3), 149–165.

Montgomery, C.M. et al. (2008) The role of partnership dynamics in determining the acceptability of condoms and microbicides. *AIDS Care* 20(6), 733–740.

Moodley, K. (2007) Microbicide research in developing countries: have we given the ethical concerns due consideration? *BMC Medical Ethics* 2007 Sep 19, 8:10.

Mystakidou, K. et al. (2009) Ethical and practical challenges in implementing informed consent in HIV/AIDS clinical trials in developing or resource-limited countries. *SAHARA J* 6(2), 46–57.

Newman, S.D., Andrews, J.O., Magwood, G.S. et al. (2011) Community advisory boards in community-based participatory research: a synthesis of best processes. *Preventing Chronic Disease* 8(3), A70.

Nguyen, V. K. (2010) *The Republic of Therapy: triage and sovereignty in West Africa's time of AIDS*. Duke University Press, Durham, North Carolina.

Nording, L (2014) Kenyan Doctors win landmark discrimination case. *Nature* 22nd July 2014.

Moyi Okwaro, F. and Geissler, P.W. (2015), In/dependent Collaborations: Perceptions and Experiences of African Scientists in Transnational HIV Research. *Medical Anthropology Quarterly* 29: 492–511. doi:10.1111/maq.12206

O'Neill, O. (2003) Some limits of informed consent. *Journal of Medical Ethics* 29, 4–7.

Pace, C., Talisuna, A., Wendler, D. et al. (2005) Quality of parental consent in a Ugandan malaria study. *American Journal of Public Health* 95(7), 1184–1189.

Painter, M.T., Kassamba, K.L. et al. (2004) Women's reasons for not participating in follow up visits before starting short course antiretroviral prophylaxis for prevention of mother to child transmission of HIV: qualitative interview study. *British Medical Journal* 329 (7465), 543.

Panitch, V. (2013) Exploitation, justice, and parity in international clinical research. *Journal of Applied Philosophy* 30(4), 304–318.

Parker, M. (2007) Ethnography/Ethics. *Social Science and Medicine* 65(11), 2248–2259.

Petryna, A. (2007) Clinical trials offshored: on private sector science and public health. *BioSocieties* 2(1), 21–40.

Petryna, A. (2009) *When Experiments Travel. Clinical trials and the global search for human subjects.* Princeton University Press, Princeton, New Jersey.

Pinheiro, C.P. (2008) Drug donations: what lies beneath. *Bulletin of the World Health Organization* 86(8), 580.

Pogge, T.W. (2002) Responsibilities for poverty-related ill health. *Ethics & International Affairs* 16(2), 71–79.

Prince, R.J. (2012) HIV and the moral economy of survival in an East African city. *Medical Anthropology Quarterly* 26(4), 534–556.

Prince, R.J. (2013) "Tarmacking" in the millennium city: spatial and temporal trajectories of empowerment and development in Kisumu, Kenya. *Africa: Journal of the International African Institute* 83, 582–605.

Prince, R.J. and Marsland, R. (2013) *Making and Unmaking Global Health.* Ohio University Press, Athens.

Rajan, K.S. (2005) Subjects of speculation: emergent life sciences and market logics in the United States and India. *American Anthropologist* 107(1), 19–30.

Redfield, P. (2008) Vital mobility and the humanitarian kit. In: Lakoff, A. and Collier, S. (eds.) *Biosecurity Interventions: Global Health and Security in Question.* Columbia University Press, New York, New York, pp. 147–171.

Redfield P. (2012) The unbearable lightness of expats: double binds of humanitarian mobility. *Cultural Anthropology* 27(2), 358–382.

Reubi, D. (2010) The will to modernize: a genealogy of biomedical research ethics in Singapore. *International Political Sociology* 4(2), 142–158.

Ridde, V. (2010) Per diems undermine health interventions systems and research in Africa: burying our heads in the sand. *Tropical Medicine and International Health* Doi.10.1111/j.1365-3156.2010.02607.x

Rottenburg, R. (2009) Social and public experiments and new figurations of science and politics in postcolonial Africa. *Postcolonial Studies* 12(4), 423–440.

Saha, S. and Galper, A. (2013) The ethical basis of drug donation to third world countries. *Ethics in Biology, Engineering and Medicine* 4(1), 29–46.

Samsky, A. (2011) Since we are taking the drugs: labor and value in two international drug donation programs. *Journal of Cultural Economy* 4(1), 27–43.

Samsky, A. (2012) Scientific sovereignty: how international drug donation programs reshape health, disease, and the state. *Cultural Anthropology* 27(2), 310–332.

Seth, S. (2009) Putting knowledge in its place: science, colonialism, and the postcolonial. *Postcolonial studies* 12(4), 373–388.

Shaffer, D N et al. (2006) Equitable Treatment for HIV/AIDS Clinical Trial Participants: A focus group study of patients, clinician researchers, and administrators in Western Kenya. *Journal of Medical Ethics* 32.1: 55–60.

Shretta, R., Walt, G., Brugha, R., and Snow, R.W. (2001) A political analysis of corporate drug donations: the example of Malarone in Kenya. *Health Policy and Planning* 16(2), 161–170.

Simon, C. and Mosavel, M. (2010) Community members as recruiters of human subjects: ethical considerations. *American Journal of Bioethics* 10(3), 3–11.

Simon, C. and Mosavel, M. (2011) Getting personal: ethics and identity in global health research. *Developing World Bioethics* 11(2), 82–92.

Simpson, B. (2009) 'Please give a drop of blood': blood donation, conflict and the haemato-global assemblage in contemporary Sri Lanka. *Body & Society* 15(2), 101–122.

Singh, J.A. and Mills, E.J. (2005) The abandoned trials of pre-exposure prophylaxis for HIV: what went wrong? *PLoS Medicine* 2(9): e234.

Stadler, J., et al. (2015) Adherence and the Lie in a HIV Prevention Clinical Trial. Medical Anthropology: 1-14.

Stangl, A.L. and Grossoman, C.I. (Eds.) (2013) *Global action to reduce HIV stigma and discrimination: Journal of the International Aids Society,* Volume 16, Supplement 2. Available at: http://www.jiasociety.org/index.php/jias/issue/view/1464 (accessed 25 October 2015). Includes webinar.

Strauss, R.P., Sengupta, S., Quinn, S.C., Goeppinger, J., Spaulding, C., Kegeles, S.M., and Millett, G. (2001) The role of community advisory boards: involving communities in the informed consent process. *American Journal of Public Health* 91, 1938–1943.

Street, A. (2012) Affective Infrastructure: Hospital landscapes of hope and failure. *Space and Culture* 15(1), 44–56.

Street, A. (2014) Research in the clinic. In: Street, A. *Biomedicine in an unstable place: infrastructure and personhood in a Papua New Guinean hospital.* Duke University Press, Durham, North Carolina, pp 194–222.

Sullivan, N. (2012) Enacting spaces of inequality: placing global/state governance within a Tanzanian hospital. *Space and Culture* 15(1), 57–67.

Vallely, A. et al. (2010) How informed is consent in vulnerable populations? Experience using a continuous consent process during the MDP301 vaginal microbicide trial in Mwanza, Tanzania. *BMC Medical Ethics* 2010 Jun 13, 11:10.

Vian, T., Miller, C., Themba, Z., and Bukuluki, P. (2012) Perceptions of per diems in the health sector: evidence and implications. *Health Policy and Planning,* 10 (1093), 1–10.

Wendland, C. L. (2008) Research, therapy, and bioethical hegemony: the controversy over perinatal AZT trials in Africa. *African Studies Review* 51(3), 1–23.

Wendland, C. L. (2010) *A Heart for the Work: Journeys through an African medical school.* University of Chicago Press, Chicago, Illinois.

Whyte, S. R. (2014) Therapeutic research in low-income countries: studying trial communities. *Archives of Disease in Childhood* 99(11) 1029-1032.

Will, C.M. (2011) Mutual benefit, added value? Doing research in the National Health Service. *Journal of Cultural Economy* 4(1), 11–26.

INDEX OF CASE STUDIES

LEARNING OBJECTIVES

Researcher/participant relationships

Community and family relationships

Institutional relationships

Staff relationships

CASE STUDIES BY KEYWORD

Employment issues

Friendship

Gender

Government

ABOUT THE CONTRIBUTORS

Philister Adhiambo Madiega has worked in community engagement and conducted fieldwork activities for a transnational medical research station in East Africa for more than eight years. She is currently a community liaison officer working on several major HIV clinical trials. Prior to this she worked for several years in ethnographic field studies. She holds a Masters in Public Health from the London School of Hygiene and Tropical Medicine, where she wrote her dissertation on the experiences of HIV care and treatment support staff.

Gemma Aellah is Research Officer at the Royal Anthropological Institute, UK, where she is committed to promoting collaborative research practices and innovative ways of encouraging public engagement with anthropology. She is also a social anthropologist who has carried out extensive fieldwork on medical research practices, first within UK psychiatric clinical trials and then in both urban and rural East Africa. Her doctoral research at the London School of Hygiene and Tropical Medicine is a fine-grained ethnography of a group of villages in East Africa, exploring the place of transnational medical research activities in the everyday lives of the researchers, participants and the wider community.

Birgitte Bruun is a Postdoctoral Fellow in the Department of Social Anthropology, University of Copenhagen. She has carried out anthropological studies of health and medicine, interspersed with project consultancies, in West and Southern Africa and Asia for almost 20 years. She has extensive experience with cross-disciplinary teamwork in international public health settings, from in the field, to at a national policy-making level. Her PhD project explored lay engagement in transnational medical research projects in southern Africa.

Tracey Chantler is a Research Fellow at the London School of Hygiene and Tropical Medicine, and has been involved in research relating to vaccine and immunization for the past 15 years. She has a background in nursing, and experience of coordinating community health and immunization programmes in Haiti, which included supervising and training community health workers. Her research experience spans paediatric clinical vaccine trials; qualitative and mixed methods research on the delivery of vaccine programmes in the UK; vaccine trial participation; public engagement; acceptance of new vaccines; and longer-term ethnographic fieldwork related to community engagement, vaccine trials and ethics in East Africa.

Luisa Enria is a Research Fellow at the London School of Hygiene and Tropical Medicine. She is currently working as a social scientist on an Ebola vaccine trial in Sierra Leone

Paul Wenzel Geissler teaches social anthropology at the University of Oslo, and works part-time at the University of Cambridge. He has worked in East Africa for over 20 years. He first studied zoology and conducted field research in medical parasitology, before converting to social anthropology. His current research concerns the ethnography of medical science, initially focusing on questions of political economy and ethics, and more recently on history, memory and the relations between temporality and the material. Among his recent books are *The Land is Dying* (Berghahn, 2011) with Ruth Prince, and *Para-states and Medical Science: Making African Global Health* (Duke, 2015).

Ann H. Kelly is a Senior Lecturer in Global Health in the Department of Social Science, Health & Medicine, at King's College, London. Her work focuses on the practices of medical research and scientific production, with special attention to the built environment, material artefacts, and experimentation practices in East and West Africa. She has been involved in a number of collaborations with scientists, health economists, and policy experts, in the UK and around the world.

Shelley Lees is a Senior Lecturer in the Department of Global Health and Development at the London School of Hygiene and Tropical Medicine. Over the past 15 years she has conducted research studies on maternal health, HIV, HPV, and gender-based violence in East Africa. Much of her research has been conducted in the context of randomized control trials where, as an anthropologist, she has been able to explore how women utilize technologies or interventions (such as microbicides, participatory training, microfinance) to address adversity. She is also currently leading anthropological research into a trial in West Africa involving Ebola, exploring both potential concerns and rumours which could impact on participation, and the ethical conduct of the trial.

Johnson A. Ondiek is – as well as an artist – a Study Coordinator and clinical officer with over ten years' experience in HIV Research and Prevention, at the Research and Public Health Collaboration programme, KEMRI / CDC, Kenya. Prior to this he spent three years as a clinical officer, working for the Kenyan Ministry of Health in HIV care.

Ferdinand Moyi Okwaro is a sociocultural anthropologist with more than ten years' experience in global health research in sub-Saharan Africa. He has designed and conducted research on a wide range of topics, including his most recent Wellcome Trust-funded project on the ethics of collaboration in transnational medical research in sub-Saharan Africa. His previous work includes studies on ritual healing, reproductive health, infectious diseases such as malaria and HIV/AIDS, social marketing, and participatory rural appraisal. He is an 'engaged anthropologist', seeking to demonstrate how anthropology can contribute to solving real-world problems. He is currently working on a project on the practice of collaboration in East Africa, funded by the Norwegian Research Council.

Francesca Raphaely is a communications and copy-editing specialist with a passion for creative writing. She studied English at the University of Cambridge, and holds a Masters in the Social Anthropology of Development from the School of Oriental and African Studies, University of London, where her dissertation explored developing news cultures in Vietnam. Her employment background is in the voluntary and community sector, working for a range of UK and international charities in communications and project management roles, and she has lived and worked in Vietnam.

John Vulule, the advisor on this workbook, is a Chief Research Officer at the Kenya Medical Research Institute (KEMRI) based at the Centre for Global Health Research. He has a research career record spanning over two and a half decades. Over the past 15 years he has been involved in research management of a Centre with a very diverse research portfolio, ranging from non-communicable diseases, infectious diseases, and even programmatic work. He is the Principal Investigator on several projects and has previously served as the Principal Investigator for the KEMRI and CDC Collaboration, a unique and multi-faceted platform where research impact can be measured.

www.ingramcontent.com/pod-product-compliance
Lightning Source LLC
LaVergne TN
LVHW082121200926
848484LV00008B/1988